THE K

for Physioth...

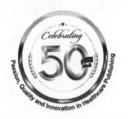

THE KNEE
for Physiotherapists

Monalisa Pattnaik MPT

Assistant Professor
Department of Physiotherapy
Swami Vivekanand National Institute of
Rehabilitation Training and Research (SVNIRTAR)
Cuttack, Odisha, India

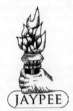

JAYPEE

JAYPEE BROTHERS MEDICAL PUBLISHERS
The Health Sciences Publisher
New Delhi | London | Panama

Jaypee Brothers Medical Publishers (P) Ltd

Headquarters
Jaypee Brothers Medical Publishers (P) Ltd
4838/24, Ansari Road, Daryaganj
New Delhi 110 002, India
Phone: +91-11-43574357
Fax: +91-11-43574314
Email: jaypee@jaypeebrothers.com

Overseas Offices

J.P. Medical Ltd
83 Victoria Street, London
SW1H 0HW (UK)
Phone: +44 20 3170 8910
Fax: +44 (0)20 3008 6180
Email: info@jpmedpub.com

Jaypee-Highlights Medical Publishers Inc
City of Knowledge, Bld. 235, 2nd Floor
Clayton, Panama City, Panama
Phone: +1 507-301-0496
Fax: +1 507-301-0499
Email: cservice@jphmedical.com

Jaypee Brothers Medical Publishers (P) Ltd
Bhotahity, Kathmandu, Nepal
Phone: +977-9741283608
Email: kathmandu@jaypeebrothers.com

Website: www.jaypeebrothers.com
Website: www.jaypeedigital.com

© 2019, Jaypee Brothers Medical Publishers

The Knee for Physiotherapists

First Edition: **2019**

ISBN 978-93-5270-267-1

Printed at Rajkamal Electric Press, Plot No. 2, Phase-IV, Kundli, Haryana.

Dedicated to

Guruji Budhabapa,
Without your love, I would
not have been able to achieve my goal.

Preface

The Knee for Physiotherapists is written to meet the needs of the students, teachers and clinicians. A keen attempt has been made to make the book useful. The initial chapters of the book cover the basic anatomy and the biomechanics of the knee. For appropriate planning of the physiotherapy management, evaluation and assessment is the key. Therefore, this book has been written in such a way that it may equip the students with basic knowledge of evaluation and assessment. Almost all the knee problems related to physiotherapy such as soft tissue injuries, arthritic conditions, etc. are included in this book, so it will be convenient to get the overall physiotherapy management of the mechanical knee problems in one book. I have tried my best to include as much evidence as possible. I hope this book will provide useful guidance to the students, teachers and clinicians alike. I would like to receive feedback and modification from the readers. Any suggestions towards its further improvement will be thankfully acknowledged and incorporated in the next edition.

Monalisa Pattnaik

Acknowledgments

I would like to thank Miss Shalini Singhal and all the students of MPT (2014-2016) of SVNIRTAR for their invaluable source of information and help for the photography.

Contents

Chapter 1

Anatomy and Biomechanics of the Knee

ANATOMY OF KNEE JOINT

The knee joint is the largest and possibly the most complex synovial joint in the body. It is a combination of three articulations, one sellar (gliding) joint between the femur and patella and two condylar joints between the two longest lever arms of the body, i.e. medial and lateral condyles of femur and tibia and bears a majority of body weight.

Osseous Components (Fig. 1.1)

Distal end of femur consists of two large condyles, separated posteriorly by very deep intercondylar notch and anteriorly by patellar

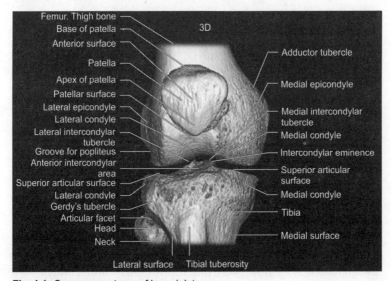

Fig. 1.1: Osseous anatomy of knee joint.
(*Source:* Micheau A, Hoa D. Anatomy of the knee (MRI)—atlas of the human body using cross-sectional imaging. 2008).

groove in which the patella glides. The anterior condylar surface is referred to as the trochlear surface (Fig. 1.1). The articular cartilage extends farther proximally on the anterior surface of the lateral condyle of femur than the medial condyle to articulate with the patella, which usually tracks upward and laterally during knee extension by the resultant quadriceps force vector.

The medial condyle extends farther distally than the lateral, so that in extension of the knee, the femur and tibia form a valgus angle of about 10°. Both condyles have epicondyles extending from their sides. Above the medial epicondyle of femur lies the adductor tubercle to which the hip adductors are inserted. Lateral condyle extends considerably farther anteriorly than the medial condyle to prevent lateral dislocation of patella caused by horizontal component of quadriceps pull. Medial condyle angles backward and medially whereas the lateral condyle lies in the sagittal plane.

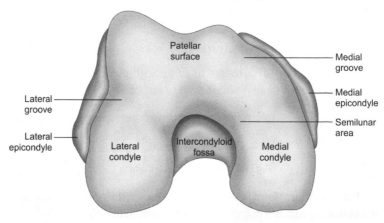

Fig. 1.2: Condyles of femur.

Looking medially or laterally, the condyles do not describe part of a circle but rather their radius gradually reduces from anterior to posteriorly. Medial condyle is longer anteroposteriorly with a more gradual change in radius, whereas the smaller lateral condyle tends to flatten sooner as one follows the curvature from back to front (Fig. 1.2).

The upper end of tibia consists of two large condyles with the articular surfaces facing upward for the articulation with femur. They are angulated 5–10° downward anteroposteriorly. Both condyles are offset posteriorly to overhang the shaft. The medial tibial condyle is larger than the lateral. The superior articulating surface of medial condyle is concave in all directions, whereas the lateral condyle is actually convex anteroposteriorly. Posterolaterally on the inferior aspect of lateral tibial condyle presents an articular facet for fibula. At the front, both the tibial condyles unite to form tibial tuberosity into which patellar tendon inserts. Superiorly medial and lateral intercondylar tubercles or eminences lie in the intercondylar area between the condyles.

Patella is a triangular shape largest sesamoid bone in the body with its apex pointing inferiorly, embedded in the back of the quadriceps tendon. It is situated in front of the lower end of femur about 1 cm above the knee joint (Fig. 1.3).

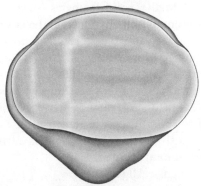

Fig. 1.3: Patellar articular surface.

Patellofemoral joint is a sellar joint between the patella and femur. It is considered one of the most complex joints in the human body from the biomechanical point of view. The posterior aspect of the patella particularly the median vertical ridge is coated with thick cartilage (4–5 mm thick) which is the thickest in the body. On either side of the median ridge, there are two biconcave facets, the lateral, related to the lateral aspect of the trochlea; the medial related to the medial aspect. It is further subdivided by a low oblique ridge into a main facet and an accessory facet, which lies at the superomedial angle and is related to the medial edge of the intercondylar fossa during extreme flexion. Normally, the small medial facet is non-articulatory. In lateral patellar tracking dysfunction, it becomes articulating giving rise to anterior knee pain. Patella provides leverage for quadriceps tendon, protects internal structures of the knee joint anteriorly against direct trauma, gives cosmetic rounded contour to the joint instead of flat appearance and provides an intermediate link of cartilage cells, lowering friction that occurs from cartilage to cartilage rather than from cartilage to tendon.

The stabilizing actions of the medial and lateral retinaculae, that tether the patella from either side to guide it into the trochlear groove in the early phase of knee flexion, are related to the specific structures, the medial patellofemoral ligament (MPFL), and the fibers originating from the iliotibial tract laterally. The quadriceps muscles have different orientations, and converge onto the patella not only from side-to-side but also posteriorly, thus pulling the patella from the anterior aspect of trochlea.[1]

The lateral retinaculum is two layers; the superficial oblique retinaculum and a deep transverse retinaculum. The superficial oblique is the culmination of the interdigitating of the patellar tendon, the VL group and the iliotibial band (ITB). The IT band originates from the fascia lata and the gluteus maximus with its attachment on the femur and Gerdy's tubercle on the anterior proximal tibia.[2]

The medial retinaculum is much thinner than the lateral retinaculum and consists of three ligaments beneath the retinaculum;
1. Medial patellofemoral ligament
2. Medial patellomeniscal ligament
3. Medial patellotibial ligament.[3]

MPFL has been demonstrated to contribute 60% of the force that opposes lateral displacement of the patella, and MPFL injury results in an approximately 50% reduction in the force needed to dislocate the patella laterally with the knee extended.

The height of the patella with respect to the trochlear groove plays a decisive role in correct kinematics, given that during contraction of the quadriceps the patella moves more proximally above the trochlea, in an area that lacks the side support. In the presence of patella alta, knee flexion is associated with a delay in the engagement of the patella in the trochlear groove, which increases the risk of lateral dislocation.

Relaxation of vastus medialis obliquus (VMO) at 20° of knee flexion determines a 30% reduction of lateral stability.[4]

PATELLOFEMORAL CARTILAGE

Patella cartilage exhibits distinct biochemical and mechanical properties compared with that of the tibia and femur. Femur and tibial cartilage demonstrates less in vivo deformation than patella cartilage with weight bearing loaded activities. Ex vivo measurement of cartilage mechanical properties has shown that femoral cartilage has a higher compressive aggregate modulus and lower permeability than patella cartilage. Femoral cartilage water content is lower than that of the patella, whilst its proteoglycan content is higher. Serum cartilage oligomeric matrix protein concentration, a biomarker of cartilage damage/loss, is higher in patients with tibiofemoral joint (TFJ) osteoarthritis (OA) than in patients with patellofemoral joint (PFJ) OA of similar severity. Patella cartilage volume is not related to bone mineral density.

Menisci (Fig. 1.4)

Knee joint is compound synovial joint of condylar variety. It consists of patellofemoral and tibiofemoral articulations.

Medial and lateral menisci are fibrocartilaginous structure that deepens the tibial articulating surfaces.

The primary function of the meniscus is to transmit load across the tibiofemoral joint by increasing congruency, thereby decreasing the resultant stress placed on the articular cartilage. The menisci also play a secondary role in shock absorption, stability, lubrication, nutrition, and proprioception to the knee joint.[5]

Injuries to the menisci are recognized as a cause of significant musculoskeletal morbidity.[6]

Their peripheral attached borders are thick and convex, their free borders are thin and concave. The proximal surface are smooth and concave in contact with the articular cartilage on the femoral condyle, while their distal surface are smooth and flat, resting on the tibial articular cartilage. Medial meniscus is semicircular, forms part of a larger circle and broader posteriorly then anteriorly. Its anterior horn is attached to the anterior intercondylar area of the tibia, anterior to the attachment of the anterior cruciate ligament (ACL). Its posterior horn is attached to the posterior intercondylar area, anterior to the attachment of the posterior cruciate ligament (PCL).

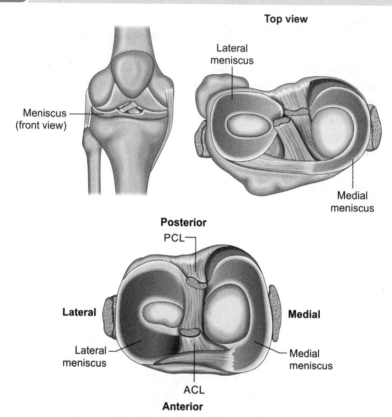

Fig. 1.4: Meniscus of the knee joint.
(PCL: posterior cruciate ligament; ACL: anterior cruciate ligament)

The lateral meniscus forms almost of a smaller circle as its both the horns are attached close to each other and is smaller and more freely moveable than the medial meniscus.

In the lateral meniscus, the anterior horn inserts on the tibia in front of the intercondylar eminence, just posterior and lateral to the ACL insertion. The posterior horn inserts to the tibia in between the insertion sites of the PCL and posterior horn of the medial meniscus and medial femoral condyle through the meniscofemoral ligaments of Wrisberg (the posterior meniscofemoral ligament) and Humphrey. (the anterior meniscofemoral ligament) (Fig. 1.4).[7]

The tendon of the popliteus separates the lateral meniscus from the fibular collateral ligament. Peripherally joint capsule is attached to the upper margin of the menisci and coronary ligament, which constitutes the inferior aspect of the joint capsule, is attached to the lower margin of the menisci. Medial collateral ligament (MCL) is attached to the medial meniscus but lateral collateral ligament (LCL) is not attached to the lateral meniscus. Therefore lateral meniscus is more mobile, whereas medial meniscus is less mobile owing to its extensive peripheral attachment. That is the reason why medial meniscus is more prone to injury.

Meniscofemoral ligament runs from the posterior aspect of the lateral meniscus to the medial femoral condyle, behind the posterior cruciate ligament. Popliteus tendon is attached to lateral meniscus and assists in posterior gliding of meniscus during knee flexion. Anteriorly both the menisci are connected by transverse ligament.

Menisci are one of the protectors of knee. It provides congruity to the articulating surfaces; absorb shock and reduces the stress. It also helps in lubrication and nutrition to the joint.

Being of fibrocartilaginous structure rather than true hyaline cartilage, they have more power of growth and healing when injured.

Capsule

Capsular ligament surrounds the knee, superiorly attaching at the margin of the femoral articular cartilage to the periphery of menisci and inferiorly from menisci to margin of the tibia, is referred as coronary ligament. Anteriorly, the capsule is absent but the patellar ligament serves as a capsule anteriorly. The fibrous capsule of the knee encloses the medial and lateral tibiofemoral joints and the patellofemoral joint. The medial capsule of the knee is very extensive, covering the entire posterior medial to anterior medial region of the knee. The medial capsule is reinforced by the MCL and medial patellar retinacular fibers, and by the expansion from the tendon of the semimembranous also known as oblique popliteal ligament. The medial capsule is further reinforced by the flat tendons of the sartorius, gracilis, and semitendinosus collectively known as the pes anserinus tendons.

The joint capsule is composed of two layers. The outer layer is fibrous connective tissue and the inner layer is synovial tissue. The outer layer is innervated with a rich supply of nerves, including mechanoreceptors and pain fibers. The mechanoreceptors sense the rate and speed of motion, the position or proprioception and have reflex connections to the muscle. Irritation or injury to the capsule can create muscle contractions, designed to protect the joint.

Synovial Membrane

The synovial membrane of the knee is the most extensive and complex in the body. The extensive synovial membrane lines the internal aspect of the fibrous capsule and is attached to the periphery of the patella and the edges of the menisci. Anterosuperiorly the synovium runs from superior aspect of patella upward underneath the quadriceps tendon then folds on itself to form a pouch—a part of the joint cavity, which provides sufficient slack in the synovium to allow knee flexion. Anteroinferiorly it lines the back of infrapatellar fat pad. At the side of the joint, the synovial membrane descends from the femur, lining the capsule as far as the menisci whose surfaces have no synovial covering. Posteriorly synovium invaginates into the intercondylar notch to pass in front of the cruciate ligament. Cruciates are intracapsular and extrasynovial. Posterior to the lateral meniscus the membrane forms a subpopliteal recess between a groove on the meniscal surface and tendon of the popliteus.

Ligaments (Fig. 1.5)

The patellar ligament or ligamentum patellae are distal part of the quadriceps tendon. It is strong, thick fibrous band attached from the apex of the patella to the tibial tuberosity. The patellar ligament is anterior ligament of the knee joint.

Patellofemoral ligament is the thickening of the patellar retinaculum. It passes from the adductor tubercle of femur to the medial aspect of the patella. It often gets irritated in case of lateral patellar tracking dysfunction due to excessive tensile stress giving rise to anterior knee pain.

Medial patellofemoral ligament is the primary passive restraint to lateral patellar translation at 20° of flexion, contributing to 60% of restraining force. Medial patellomeniscal ligament and the lateral retinaculum contribute 13% and 10% of the restraint to lateral translation of the patella respectively. Superficial retinaculum consists

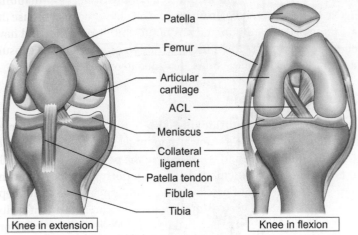

Fig. 1.5: Ligaments around knee joint.
(ACL: anterior cruciate ligament).

of fibers from vastus lateralis and iliotibial band. The deep retinaculum consists of the lateral patellofemoral ligament, the deep fibers of the iliotibial band and the lateral patello tibial ligament. They provide the passive restraint to medial translation (Fig. 1.5).

Oblique popliteal ligament is a tendinous expansion of the semi-membranosus, which strengthens the fibrous capsule posteriorly. It rises posteriorly to the medial femoral condyle and passes supero-laterally to attach to the central part of the posterior aspect of the fibrous capsule.

Arcuate popliteal ligament is a V-shaped mass of capsular fibers. It arrives from the posterior aspect of the fibular head, passes supero-medially over the tendon of the popliteus and spreads over the posterior surface of the knee joint. It strengthens the fibrous capsule posteriorly.

Collateral ligaments: Medial collateral ligament (MCL) is long and flat, attached above to the medial epicondyle of the femur and below to medial aspect of shaft of tibia about 4 cm below the joint line. It lies slightly anterior to the joint axis. It becomes taut in extension, abduction and external rotation of tibia and some of the anterior fibers become taut in flexion. It also prevents anterior displacement of tibia on femur. Its deep capsular fibers are attached to medial meniscus and compromises its mobility (Fig. 1.6).

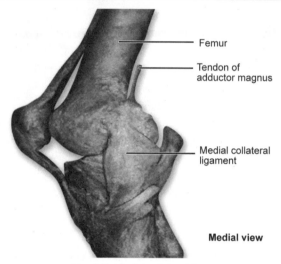

Medial view

Fig. 1.6: Medial collateral ligament.

Lateral collateral ligament is short, rounded and cord-like, attached above to the lateral epicondyle of femur and below to the head of fibula. It does not get attached to the lateral meniscus. Popliteus tendon runs underneath it, i.e. between lateral meniscus and LCL. It is covered by the biceps femoris tendon. It lies slightly posterior to the joint axis. It becomes taut in extension, adduction and external rotation of tibia (Fig. 1.7).

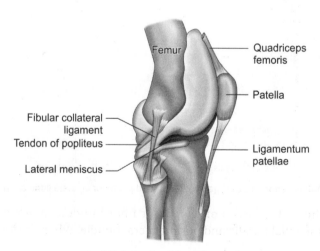

Fig. 1.7: Lateral collateral ligament.

Anterolateral ligament (ALL) originates from the anterior and distal attachment to the femoral attachment of the LCL. It spans the joint in an oblique fashion and inserts between the fibular head and Gerdy tubercle on the tibia. The ALL is a contributor to tibial internal rotation stability.[8]

Cruciate ligaments: Cruciate ligament join the femur and tibia, criss-crossing within the articular capsule of the joint but outside the synovial joint cavity. The cruciate ligaments are located in the center of the joint and cross each other obliquely like the letter "X" providing stability to the knee joint throughout the joint range of motion. They are named according to the anterior and posterior attachment to tibia (Fig. 1.8).

The anterior cruciate ligament attached medially to the anterior intercondylar area of the tibia just posterior to the attachment of the medial meniscus. It extends superiorly, posteriorly and laterally to attach to the posterior part of the medial side of the lateral condyle of the femur in the intercondylar notch. The ACL is slack when the knee is flexed and taut when it is fully extended. It checks forward displacement of tibia over femur, posterior displacement of the femur on tibia, internal rotation of tibia on femur and hyperextension of the knee joint.

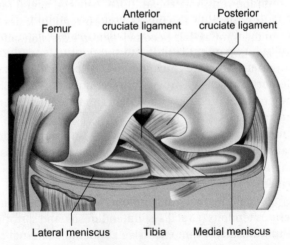

Anterior cruciate ligament | Posterior cruciate ligament | Femur | Lateral meniscus | Tibia | Medial meniscus

Fig. 1.8: Anterior cruciate ligament (ACL) and posterior cruciate ligament (PCL).

The ACL consists of two major fiber bundles, namely, the anteromedial bundle and posterolateral bundle. When the knee is extended, the posterolateral bundle is tight and the anteromedial bundle is moderately lax. As the knee is flexed, the femoral attachment of ACL becomes a more horizontal orientation, causing the AM bundle to tighten and the PL bundle to relax (Fig. 1.8).[9]

Abnormal gait after ACL reconstruction may contribute to development and/or progression of knee OA. Sagittal plane biomechanics, rather than the knee adduction moment, appear to be more relevant post-ACL reconstruction. Better understanding of sagittal plane biomechanics is necessary for optimal postoperative recovery, and to potentially prevent early onset and progression of knee OA.[10]

The PCL is stronger less oblique with some shorter fiber. It arises from the posterior intercondylar area of the tibia, passes superiorly, anteriorly and medially on the medial side of the ACL to attach to the anterior part of the lateral surface of the medial condyle of the femur in the intercondylar notch. The PCL tighten during flexion of the knee joint preventing anterior displacement of the femur on the tibia or posterior displacement of the tibia on the femur, internal rotation of tibia on femur and hyperextension of the knee. During squatting forward gliding of femur on tibia is checked by PCL and popliteus.

The lateral knee consists of numerous static and dynamic stabilizers that together provide lateral knee stability. The three primary static stabilizers include the fibular collateral ligament (FCL), popliteofibular ligament (PFL), and the popliteus tendon (PLT). Other important structures include the ITB, long and short head of biceps femoris muscle, gastrocnemius tendon, ALL, fabellofibular ligament, proximal tibiofibular ligaments and coronary ligament of the lateral meniscus.

Ligaments are reinforced by muscles. Anteriorly quadriceps tendon and patellar tendon reinforces the joint capsule. Posteriorly gastrocnemius, popliteus check external rotation and backward displacement of tibia on the femur.

Anteromedially medial patellar retinaculum and posteromedially pes anserinus tendons (Gracilis, semitendinosus, and sartorius) and semimembranosus prevent excessive abduction, external rotation and anterior displacement of tibia. It reinforces the medial collateral ligament.

Anterolaterally lateral patellar retinaculum and ITB checks excessive internal rotation tibia and reinforce the cruciates.

Posterolaterally biceps femoris tendon checks excessive internal rotation and anterior displacement of tibia. It reinforces the cruciates.

Bursae (Fig. 1.9)

Anteriorly suprapatellar pouch serves as a bursa. There are also prepatellar bursa lies in between the skin and patella, superficial infrapatellar bursa between the skin and patellar tendon and deep infrapatellar bursa between the patellar tendon and tibia.

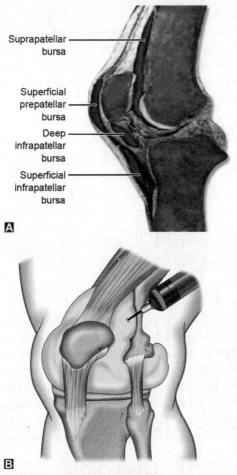

Suprapatellar bursa

Superficial prepatellar bursa

Deep infrapatellar bursa

Superficial infrapatellar bursa

A

B

Figs. 1.9A and B: Bursae around patella.

Prepatellar bursa gets inflamed with prolonged kneeling activities, referred as housemaid's knee. Posteriorly bursa between semimembranosus and medial head of gastrocnemius often communicates into the joint cavity and may become swollen secondary to joint effusion, referred as Backers cyst. Anteromedially bursae present underneath the tendons of pes anserinus and anterolaterally underneath the ITB.

Fat Pads

Large infrapatellar fat pad is situated deep to the patellar tendon in front of femoral condyles. When knee flexes it fills the anterior aspect of intercondylar notch and with knee extension it occupies patellar groove and covers the trochlear surface of the femur. Back of the fat pad is lined by the synovium and lubricates femoral articulating surface prior to contact with the tibia to facilitate the movements.

BIOMECHANICS

Medial femoral condyle extends farther distally than the lateral giving rise to slight genu valgus of about 5° to 10° with the knee in extension.

With the transcondylar axis of femur in frontal plane, patella faces slightly forward, neck of femur is directed about 20° forward because of anteversion and transmalleolar axis of the ankle is rotated outward about 25° as a result of normal external tibial torsion and long axis of foot is directed outward about 10° (Fig. 1.10).

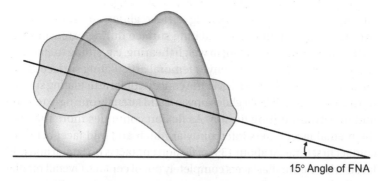

15° Angle of FNA

Fig. 1.10: Normal femoral anteversion. (FNA: femoral neck anteversion). (*Source:* APTA).

Flexion-extension of knee occurs in sagittal plane and frontal axis. 5–10° of hyperextension is limited by the tension of the posterior joint capsule and ligaments. 140–150° of flexion is limited by soft tissue approximation, i.e. contact between the calf muscles and muscles of the back of the thigh. Extension is referred as close packed position. Valgus in extension disappears in flexion. Knee flexion-extension is polycentric, the axis of movement shifts backward along a curved centroid as knee moves from extension into flexion (Fig. 1.11).

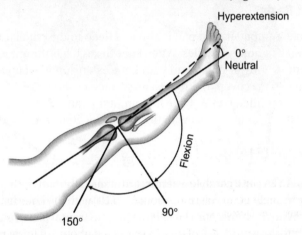

Fig. 1.11: Knee range of motion.
(*Source:* Singh AP. Knee range of motion and movements 2015. Retrieved from http://boneandspine.com).

As per the concave-convex rule, in non-weight bearing, e.g. high sitting concave tibial articulating surface glides and rolls forward over the convex femoral articulating surface during extension and backward during flexion. But in weight bearing, e.g. sitting to standing while the tibia is fixed the convex femoral articulating surface glides backward and rolls forward over the concave tibial articulating surface during extension. Patella glides upward and laterally during extension and downward during flexion. As flexion continues more than 90° the medial facet enters intercondylar notch and odd facet achieves contact first time. At about 135° of flexion contact is on lateral and odd facets whereas medial facets completely out of contact. Overall medial patellar facet normally receives most consistent contact with femoral surface whereas odd facet receives least. As patella tracks down the femur it undergoes some rotation about vertical axis called patellar tilt. It tilts medially from 0° to 30° and beyond 100°, whereas lateral tilting occurs between 20° to 100° of flexion (Figs. 1.12A and B).

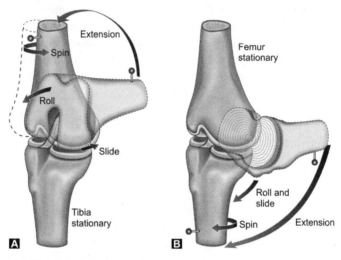

Figs. 1.12A and B: Arthrokinematic motion at knee joint.

(*Source:* Dutton's Orthopaedic examination, evaluation, and intervention, 3rd edition, Chapter 1. The Musculoskeletal System).

The anterior-posterior (AP) translation is about 5–10 mm, medial-lateral (M-L) translation is about 1–2 mm and tibiofemoral compression–distraction (C-D) is about 2–5 mm.

Tibiofemoral joint is most incongruent in flexion and becomes progressively congruent as knee extends. Tibial articulating surface remains constant throughout flexion-extension, but femoral articulating surface changes from inferior to posterior as the knee flexes from extension. In flexion, the smaller convex radius of posterior femoral condyles contact with the relatively larger radius of the tibial condyles, so the joint is most incongruent. As the knee extends femoral articulating surface progressively shifts anteriorly, the radius of curvature of which progressively increases and in extension the joint becomes most congruent.

The fibrocartilaginous menisci reduce joint incongruity. Their mobility and deformability allow them to conform to the shape of the contacting femoral surface. Anterior part of menisci is somewhat mobile whereas the posterior part is relatively fixed. Menisci move with tibia during flexion-extension and with femur during rotation. As the knee extends anterior aspect of menisci move forward over tibia allowing the larger femoral condylar surfaces to articulate; similarly during knee flexion menisci move backward over tibia allowing the smaller femoral condylar surfaces to articulate. Thus, menisci play very important role to reduce the incongruity of the tibiofemoral joint. It improves the load bearing area and reduces joint compressive stress.

There is an automatic or conjunct rotation that accompanies flexion-extension, i.e. external rotation of tibia during final 15–20° of extension and internal rotation during initial 15–20° flexion.

During lateral rotation of the tibia on the femur, the lateral condyle moves forward over the lateral tibial condyle, while the medial femoral condyle moves backward over the medial tibial condyle. The shape and orientation of medial femoral condyle contribute to such rotation, i.e. medial condyle is longer anteroposteriorly and curved and obliquely oriented whereas lateral condyle is more in sagittal plane. As knee extends the smaller diameter lateral compartment completes the movement before the larger diameter medial femoral articulating surface completes. Medial side of tibia continues to move forward along the curved medial femoral condyle, while the lateral tibial joint surface undergoes a lateral spin, resulting into external rotation of tibia on the femur to complete full extension of knee. Similarly during initial knee flexion internal tibial rotation occurs.

According to Fick, lateral rotation has a range of 40° and medial rotation a range of 30°. This range varies with the degree of knee flexion since lateral rotation attains a 32° range when the knee is flexed at 30° and 42° range when the knee is flexed at right angles.

Normal loads on articular cartilage include forces imposed by the action of muscles around the joint, as well as the force of the body weight that is transmitted through the joint. Muscle contractions that stabilize or move the joint provide a major component of the load on the articular cartilage. In addition, during normal walking, three to four times the weight of the body is transmitted through the knee joint. This force increases dramatically during maneuvers such as a deep knee bend, during which the patellofemoral joint is subjected to a load 9–10 times the body's weight. Although articular cartilage is an excellent shock absorber, it is only 3–6 mm thick at maximum, and thus provides limited joint protection. Thus, the joint must have other protective mechanisms, which include the action of muscles around the joint and the protection of the subchondral bone and the shock-absorbing functions of the synovial fluid. The surrounding muscles play a key role in imposing forces on the joint and also act as shock absorbing mechanisms. Muscles store energy when stretched during joint motion, and they dissipate or absorb this energy rather than transferring it to the vulnerable joint structures. Thus, adequate muscle strength and bulk are protective to the joint. In addition, rapid neuromuscular (reflex) responses also serve to shield the joint from unexpected forces.

During walking, the ground reaction force vector passes medial to the knee joint center, creating an external adduction moment about the knee. The adduction moment determines the load distribution across the medial compartment almost 2.5 times that of the lateral. Varus knee malalignment, which typically accompanies a loss of joint space in medial TFJ OA, serves only to increase the moment arm of the force vector, thereby increasing the adduction moment (Fig. 1.13).

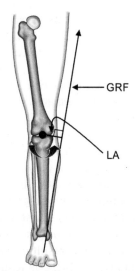

Fig. 1.13: Ground reaction force (GRF) at knee joint.

(*Source:* Rozen N. Biomechanical aspects of knee osteoarthritis and Apos Therapy. http://www.apostherapy.co.uk).

Q-angle is the upwardly faced angle that formed by the bisection of lines joining anterior superior iliac spine and midpoint of patella, and joining tibial tuberosity and midpoint of patella. Normally Q-angle is 13–18°, about 13° in males and 18° in females (Fig. 1.14). It reduces to 8–10° in sitting with quadriceps contraction in full knee extension and becomes 0° in sitting with knee flexed to 90°.

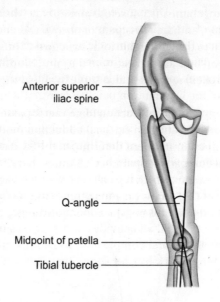

Fig. 1.14: Q-angle.

(*Source:* Marra D. Q-angle, Patella and Quads. 2013. https://www.yogatuneup.com).

The Q-angle is a clinical measure of lower limb alignment that represents the resultant force orientation of the four components of the quadriceps muscles acting on the patella in the frontal plane. The resultant of quadriceps muscle force in the frontal plane can be determined by the following way. The direction of quadriceps muscle pull is from the midpoint of patella to anterior superior iliac spine (ASIS) and that of the ligamentum patellae is from the midpoint of patella to tibial tuberosity. Their resultant can be determined by the law of parallelogram (Fig. 1.14). The resultant is that diagonal that emerges from the midpoint of patella, which faces upward and outward, i.e. with active quadriceps contraction patella tracks upward and outward. Lateral subluxation of patella is prevented by anterior prominence of lateral femoral condyle, deep patellar groove and dynamically by the force of contraction of VMO. This laterally directed force vector results in the lateral patella facet receiving 60% more force than the medial facet.

The PFJ reaction force is the measure of the compression of the patella against the femur. During weight-bearing activities, it is the vector summation of the quadriceps muscle and patellar ligament forces. The resultant of quadriceps muscle force and patellar ligament force in the sagittal plane can be determined by the following way. The direction of quadriceps muscle pull is from the midpoint of patella to ASIS and that of the ligamentum patellae is from the midpoint of patella to tibial tuberosity. Their resultant can be determined by the law of parallelogram, i.e. completing the parallelogram in the sagittal plane (Fig. 1.15). The resultant is that diagonal that emerges from the midpoint of patella, which faces backward. As knee moves from extension to flexion the resultant progressively increases, i.e. with increasing knee flexion patellofemoral compressive force increases. That is the reason why persons with patellofemoral degenerative joint disease are advised to avoid all activities and exercises that involve knee bending. Patellofemoral compressive force for walking $=1.5 \times$ BW, for stair climbing $= 3.3 \times$ BW, for squatting $= 8$–$9 \times$ BW.

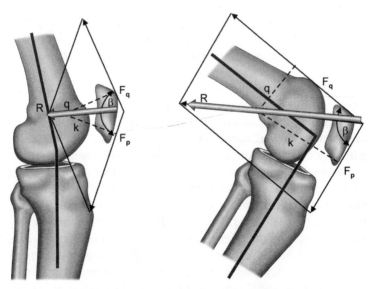

Fig. 1.15: Forces at patellofemoral joint.
(*Source:* Biomechanics of patellofemoral rehabilitation).

An important contributor to the distribution of the PFJ reaction force is the alignment and motion of the patella with the femoral trochlea. Patella alignment relies on passive (osseous configuration and soft tissue restraints) and active (medial and lateral quadriceps) structures. The osseous anatomical anomalies most likely to affect the alignment and motion of the patella are a shallow femoral trochlea groove depth and patella alta. Soft tissue restraints such as medial and lateral retinacula: particularly the two distal expansions of the ITB, the joint capsule and ligaments contribute to maintain patella alignment. The quadriceps muscle, VMO, the more distal portion of the medial quadriceps, and the vastus lateralis are essential for optimal patella alignment. Normally, the iliotibial tract moves posteriorly over the lateral femoral condyle when the knee is flexed beyond 30°. Fulkerson and Hunger ford states that the lateral retinacular bands are drawn posteriorly along with the ITB on knee flexion. This causes progressive tilting of the patella laterally if the medial static stabilizers are stretched or the dynamic stabilizers (VMO) are weak. Balance of the medial and lateral static and dynamic stabilizers is necessary for proper alignment of the patella for pain free function. If the lateral structures become shortened, there will be excessive lateral translatory force exerted on the patella, causing lateral patellar compression syndrome and possibly subluxation. PFJ malalignment leads to increased contact pressure on an individual facet, e.g. lateral tilt of the patella leads to increased contact pressure on the lateral facet.

Lower limb alignment may affect patella tracking by altering the relative position of the femoral trochlea and changing the tension in soft tissues. Notably, experimentally-induced femoral internal rotation or tibial external rotation have been associated with increased lateral patellar tilt and rotation and increased lateral PFJ pressure.

Patella is fixed to the tibia via the patellar tendon. During external rotation, when the tibial tuberosity moves laterally, the patellar tendon functions to pull on the distal pole of the patella laterally and rotates the superior aspect of the patella medially about the center of the patella increasing the Q-angle and lateral PFJ pressure.

Internal rotation is coupled with subtalar joint pronation, while external rotation is coupled with subtalar joint supination. Abnormal pronation results in a rotatory strain on the soft tissues of the lower extremity. Excessive tibia internal rotation caused by abnormal subtalar joint pronation would actually decrease the Q angle and the lateral forces acting on the patella. Tiberio described excessive pronation would affect normal patellofemoral joint function. He postulated that to achieve extension in midstance, the tibia must externally rotate relative to the femur to ensure adequate motion for the screw home mechanism. To compensate for the lack of tibial external rotation caused by the failure of the foot to resupinate, the femur would have to internally rotate on the tibia such that the tibia was in relative external rotation. In turn, excessive internal rotation of the femur would move the patella medially, with respect to ASIS and the tibial tuberosity thereby increasing the Q angle and the lateral component of the quadriceps muscle.

The range of patellofemoral total contact pressure with respect to tibial rotation was 0.81–1.23 MPa, 1.04–1.49 MPa, 0.95–1.20 MPa, and 1.01–1.32 MPa at 0°, 30°, 60° and 90° respectively. The total contact pressures were relatively similar at all knee flexion angles except 0°, where they were the lowest. At each knee flexion, 15° of external tibial rotation had the highest pressure. Tibial rotation decreased the in situ strain of the contralateral side of the retinaculum with respect to the direction of tibial rotation, often accompanied by an increase in the in situ strain of the ipsilateral side of the retinaculum.

With internal femoral rotation, the lateral articular surface of the trochlea impinges upon the lateral articular facets of the retropatellar surface, in essence pushing the patella medially. At the same time, the peripatellar retinaculum, whose predominant attachments are at the femoral epicondyles, rotates along with the femur and "pulls" it along it. With external rotation of the femur, the medial articular surface of the trochlea impinges upon the medial articular facets of the retropatellar surface, pushing the patella laterally.

Resting position of knee is 25° of flexion, close packed position is full extension, and capsular pattern is limitation of flexion beyond 90° and limitation of terminal 20° extension. Range of motion (ROM) required for some common activities of daily livings are for normal human locomotion stance phase –21° of flexion, swing phase 67° flexion; stair climbing requires 83° of flexion and sitting to standing and standing to sitting requires 83° of flexion.

Compressive forces in dynamic knee joint are 2–3 times body weight in normal gait, 5–6 times body weight in running and stair climbing. The menisci assume 40–60% of the imposed load. If the menisci are removed, magnitude of average load per unit area on articular cartilage nearly doubles on the femur and is 6–7 times greater on the tibial condyle. Elimination of the physiological valgus angle at knee will increase compression on medial meniscus by 25%.

Pathomechanics

With excessive genu valgum, there is compression on the lateral aspect of the joint and distraction on the medial aspect. The weight bearing shifts to lateral compartment. Increased loading over time will give rise to lateral compartment degenerative joint disease. There will be excessive tensile stress over the MCL and capsule. There develop secondary foot pronation and foot pain. Increased Q-angle will give rise to lateral patellar tracking dysfunction and anterior knee pain. With excessive genu varum, there is compression on the medial aspect of the joint and distraction on the lateral aspect. The weight-bearing shifts to medial compartment. Increased loading over time will give rise to medial compartment degenerative joint disease. There will be excessive tensile stress over the LCL and capsule. There develop secondary foot supination.

With valgus stress, there is tension over the medial aspect of the knee joint leading to stretching of MCL. Depending on the amount of force, there will be variable degrees of MCL sprain. With severe sprain, there will be damage to medial joint capsule. If the force becomes more, there will be injury to medial meniscus to which the deep fibers of MCL gets attached. If the force further exceeds, there will be injury to ACL. The conditions in which all these three ligaments are damaged are known as triad of O'Donoghue. Similar type of injury on the medial aspect of the knee joint is uncommon as both the medial sides are well protected.

Normally peak weight-bearing force is transmitted at mid-stance or loading phase of the gait cycle, during which the knee remains about 10° flexion, near closed pack position where tibiofemoral contact area is more; so the load is less. In case of capsular contracture or knee flexion deformity one has to load the joint in more flexed position, where tibiofemoral contact area is reduced than normal; so the loading will be increased. It will predispose or precipitate degeneration of tibiofemoral joint. That is the reason why full extension must be restored before restoration of flexion range of motion and weight bearing in bend knee should be discouraged.

Rotatory dysfunctions: Normally external rotation of tibia in non-weight bearing or internal rotation of femur in weight bearing occurs during terminal knee extension and internal rotation of tibia in non-weight bearing or external rotation of femur in weight bearing occurs during initial flexion. Full extension is possible in the absence of normal rotation, but at the expense of deformation of articular tissues, i.e. sprain meniscus. Extension without rotation or with abnormal rotation put stress over the meniscus giving rise to injury. Rotation at complete extension is not possible, but forced rotation put stress over the meniscus. In extension the menisci are at their extreme forward position, with rotation either of the menisci tends to move forward and the other tends to move back. There will be excessive stress over the former leading to injury. Similarly in hyperflexed knee, i.e. in squatting, where the menisci are at their extreme posterior position, rotation in either direction will tend to move one of the menisci backward and the other forward. The one which tends to move back will have excessive stress and gets injured because it cannot move further back.

In normal standing position feet faces outward, knees forward with the hips in neutral positions. In case of femoral anteversion, with the hips in neutral positions knees face inward (squinting patellae) and toes pointing inward (in-toeing). With internal rotation of hip to maintain it in neutral position, there develops genu valgus and pronated foot. Some may develop compensatory external tibial torsion. Similarly in case of femoral retroversion patellae face outward with genu varum and out-toeing with foot supination.

Anterior to posterior displacement of tibial as occurs in case of falling on the knees or due to dash board injury, where the car-board dashes over the upper end of tibia displacing it backward results in injury PCL. Similar type of injury to damage ACL is uncommon. Forced internal rotation may result in isolated injury of ACL.

Hyperextension injury results in tearing of posterior capsule followed by anterior cruciate ligament and then posterior cruciate ligament.

REFERENCES

1. Andrew A, et al. Current concepts on anatomy and biomechanics of patellar stability. Sports Medicine and Arthroscopy Review. 2007;15(2):48-56.
2. McConnell J. Rehabilitation and nonoperative treatment of patellar instability. Sports Med Arthrosc. 2007;15:95-104.
3. Waryasz GR, et al. Patellofemoral pain syndrome [PFPS]: a systematic review of anatomy and potential risk factors. Dyn Med. 2008;7:9.
4. Zaffagnini, et al. Patellofemoral anatomy and biomechanics: current concepts. Joints. 2013;1(2): 15-20.
5. Englund M, Guermazi A, Lohmander LS. The menisci in knee osteoarthritis. Rheum Dis Clin North Am. 2009;35:579-90.
6. Fox AJ, Bedi A, Rodeo SA. The basic sience of human knee menisci: structure, composition and function. Sports Health. 2012;4:340-51.
7. Mckeon BP, Bono JV, Richmond JC. Knee Arthroscopy, New York, NY: Springer Science and Business Media; 2009.
8. Pomajzil, et al. A review of the anterolateral ligament of the knee: current knowledge regarding its incidence, anatomy, biomechanics, and surgical dissection Arthroscopy. 2015;32 (3):583-91.
9. Petersen W, Zantop T. Anatomy of the anterior cruciate ligament with regard to its two bundles. Clinical Orthopedics and Related Research. 2007; 454: 35-47.
10. Hart, et al. Knee kinematics and joint moments during gait following anterior cruciate ligament reconstruction: a systematic review and meta-analysis. Br J Spotrs Med. 2015;50(10):597-612.

Chapter 2

Evaluation

Traumatic lesions may be experienced by the athletes as well as by the more sedentary individual. Degenerative arthritis occurs in elderly individual. Overuse fatigue syndromes may affect at any age group. The approach to evaluation of knee disorders may be sufficiently flexible to accommodate such a broad spectrum of disorders.

HISTORY

Mode of onset: Traumatic lesions are sudden in onset. Find out the mechanism of injury. Valgus-external rotation injuries are the most common traumatic knee disorders injuring medial collateral ligament, medial joint capsule, medial meniscus and anterior cruciate ligament (ACL).

History of swelling: Whether the swelling develops immediately after the injury within some minutes to hours or gradually over a period of hours to days? Immediate joint swelling is hemarthrosis, which occurs due to injury of some highly vascular structure. It develops within some minutes to hours, quite tense with gross limitation of joint range of motion (ROM). It is very painful. Joint effusion develops slowly over a period of hours to days. Fluctuation test is positive, joint range of motion is limited in capsular pattern with muscle spasm end feel. In case of hemarthrosis, X-rays should be done to rule out intra-articular fracture before any intervention.

History of pain: Knee joint is supplied by L3 to S2 segments. Antero-medial aspect of knee is supplied by L3, which does not extend much below the knee. So pain from the pathology involving anteromedial structures of knee does not refer below the knee, i.e. pain is always localized over the structure involved. Posterior aspect of knee is supplied by S1 and S2. Pain from joint effusion is often experienced on the back of the knee, which may refer distally up to the foot. Pain from lumbosacral pathology radiates to the knee or that from hip pathology may refer to the front of the knee. Anteromedial pain localized to joint line of sudden onset is meniscus or collateral ligament sprain. Medial knee pain of traumatic origin following valgus and rotatory strain is medial capsule-ligamentous injury.

Severity of pain is proportional to severity of injury. Pain is well localized in case of mild injury involving the superficial structure. Pain is diffused, not well localized, in case of moderate injury with joint effusion. In case of severe injury with complete rupture of the capsule the effusion fluid escapes out of the joint cavity. So, there is no joint swelling, no limitation of motion and pain is not proportional to the severity of injury.

Impairment of function: Following injury there is swelling and pain. Loss of function is proportional to the severity of swelling and pain. In case of complete rupture, pain is proportionately less as no intact nerve ending is left. In the absence of swelling and pain one can perform activities. Later on as muscle spasm develops to guard the instability some pain is experienced and movements get limited. At such stage, it is difficult to properly assess the client. Evaluation should be done following prolong ice application or medication or under anesthesia. There are evidences of highly motivated sports persons able to get up unaided and resumed play following complete rupture in competitive games.

Gradual nontraumatic onset: Age, occupation, nature of duty, change in nature of duty, change in gadget or environmental factors, etc. should be noted. Sedentary over-weight persons are prone to develop degenerative joint disease or fatigue over use syndrome.

❑ Does the knee click, grind, grate or pop, catch?[1]
❑ Does the knee ever locked, buckled or given way? If so, under which circumstances?
❑ Is stair climbing, ascending/descending a problem?
❑ Is it possible to run? What is the effect of turning, running backward, running with sudden stop and change in directions quickly?

Elderly person with knee flexion deformity finding difficulty to squat, climb stairs, walk, stand from sitting, etc. with crepitus during movements are characteristic features of tibiofemoral degenerative joint disease. Nontraumatic anterior knee pain of gradual onset, worsen on descending/ascending stairs and prolonged sitting with knee bend is characteristic features of patellofemoral degenerative joint disease.

History of locking and giving way is the characteristic features of torn meniscus. History of giving way and pain while turning away from the involved side is the characteristic features of torn medial collateral ligament (MCL). History of giving way during descending steps or squatting or running with sudden stop is the characteristic features of torn posterior cruciate ligament (PCL). History of giving way during running is the characteristic features of torn ACL. Catching is more typical with either extensor mechanism disorder (maltracking of patella) or small meniscal tear.[1]

PHYSICAL EXAMINATION

I. Observation

Gait, functional activities such as stair climbing, running, sudden change in direction, sitting and getting up, squatting, jumping, etc.

II. Inspection

A. In Standing

1. *Frontal alignment:* The patient is viewed from the front and from the back. Vertical and horizontal asymmetries in frontal plane detected by determining positions of navicular tubercle, medial and lateral malleoli, heels, fibular head, popliteal folds, tibial tuberosities, tibial and femoral condyles, gluteal folds, greater trochanter (GT), anterior superior iliac spine (ASIS), posterior superior iliac spine (PSIS), iliac crest, etc.

    Vertical disparities are determined by checking bilateral symmetry of two identical structures from a reference, in standing ground is taken as the reference. Horizontal disparities are determined by checking two identical landmarks from a reference, bony landmark on the body midline such as manubrium sternum, xiphoid, umbilicus or symphysis pubis is taken as the reference or plumb line dropped from body midline is taken as the reference.
    - Leg length differences
    - Genu valgus, varus, tibia valga, vara

2. *Transverse rotary alignment:* The patient is viewed from the front. Intermalleolar line is normally rotated to 25 to 30° outward from the frontal plane.

   Tibial tubercle should be in line with the midline or lateral half of patella. Patellae faces straight forward, patellae facing inward is referred as squinting patellae, which is the characteristic of femoral anteversion or external tibial torsion.

   Normally length of patella tendon is almost equal to length of patella (1.2:1),[1] higher ridding patella is referred as patella alta (ratio greater than 1.2:1) and low lying patella is referred as patella baja, length of patella tendon is lesser than length of patella.

   Normally Q-angle is 13–18°, 13° in male and 18° in female. In sitting with quadriceps contraction in full extension of knee Q-angle reduces to 8–10° and in sitting with the knee flexed to 90° Q-angle vanishes.

3. *Anteroposterior alignment*: The patient is viewed from the side. A plumb line is dropped from the mastoid process or lateral side of the shoulder joint to check spinal lordosis/kyphosis, knee flexion/genu recurvatum. Normally, it should pass through the tip of GT, slight anterior to knee, about 1 cm anterior to lateral malleolus.

B. Sitting

1. *Femoropatellar alignment*: Patella faces straight forward with the inferior pole level with tibiofemoral joint line. A small, high ridding, outward facing patella may predispose to lateral patellar tracking dysfunction. A laterally facing patella may suggest genu valgus.

2. *Tibiofemoral alignment*: Tibial tubercle lines up with the midline or lateral half of patella. A tubercle that lies too far medially indicates posteromedial capsular tightness or tight healed cruciate ligament. A tubercle that lies too far laterally indicates laxity of posteromedial capsule or MCL.

C. Supine

1. All goniometric measurement performs.

2. *Leg length measurement:* Apparent limb lengths are measured by positioning both the lower limbs parallel to each other and aligned

along the trunk. Measurement is taken from the xiphoid/umbilicus or symphysis pubis to the tip of medial malleolus or heel.

3. For true limb length square or level the pelvis; to level both ASIS, if the affected side is down, abduct and hyperabduct till both ASIS get leveled. Now adduct it till the ASIS tends to move down. Position opposite limb in symmetrical position. Measurement is taken from the ASIS to the tip of medial malleolus or heel. If the affected side is up, adduct and hyperadduct till both ASIS get leveled. Now abduct it till the ASIS tends to move up. Position opposite limb in symmetrical position. Measurement is taken from the ASIS to the tip of medial malleolus or heel.

4. Segmental limb length can be measured in crook lying position with hips flexed to 45° and knees to 90°. Femoral length is measured from tip of GT to lateral femoral condyle. Tibial length measurement is taken from medial tibial flare to the tip of medial malleolus. For supratrochanteric length of femur Bryant's triangle is drawn by drawing a vertical line from the ASIS to the bed, the horizontal distance of this line from tip of GT represent the supratrochanteric length of femur.

5. In crook lying position more prominent tibial tubercle indicates Osgood-Schlatter's disease/osteochondrosis of tibial apophysis, whereas less prominent tibial tubercle indicates rupture PCL.

6. Check the skin for color, texture, moisture, and scar. Localized erythema suggests underlying inflammation. Ecchymosis on the lateral aspect of the knee results from direct blow and that on the medial aspect suggests MCL sprain. Ecchymosis on the anteromedial aspect of the knee is due to patellar dislocation. Cyanosis of lower limb is the characteristic feature of reflex sympathetic dystrophy or varicose vein or deep vein thrombosis (DVT). Erythema, smooth, glossy and wet skin indicate hypervascularity and is the characteristic feature of acute inflammation or acute reflex sympathetic dystrophy; whereas pale or cyanosed, rough, dry skin indicate hypovascularity and is characteristic feature of chronic inflammation or chronic reflex sympathetic dystrophy.

7. Check the soft tissues for wasting, swelling (generalized/localized —intra/extra-articular), contour. Generalized lower limb swelling develops following immobilization due to trauma or surgery or may be due to reflex sympathetic

dystrophy. Articular swelling manifests as swelling of the suprapatellar pouch, distention of posterior capsule and knee assumes semiflexed position. Extra-articular swelling often develop over the prepatellar bursa (housemaid's knee).

III. Movements

1. *Active movements:* Bilateral weight-bearing flexion-extension and unilateral weight-bearing flexion-extension, if not contraindicated by the recent trauma or surgery. Bilateral weight-bearing flexion-extension is checked by asking to perform squatting and note patient's willingness, range, pain, instability, crepitus, etc. For unilateral weight-bearing flexion-extension ask to perform one-legged half-squat repeatedly on the sound side followed by on the involved side to determine the strength, also note the pain, instability, crepitus, etc.

2. Active non-weight-bearing flexion-extension in supine lying by asking to perform straight leg raising, then flex the knee and again straighten it. Record the range of motion, pain, crepitus, etc. Loss of knee extension while flexion is full indicates internal derangement of the joint due to torn anterior horn of the meniscus. Limitation of terminal flexion beyond 90–100° and extension beyond 20–30° indicates capsular restriction.

3. *Quadriceps lag:* To complete last 15° of extension a 60% increase in quadriceps muscle force is required. Loss of mechanical advantages, reflex inhibition, adhesion formation, quadriceps atrophy, lengthening or inability to shorten properly, etc. may result in quadriceps lag. In supine position with a small firm pillow or block under the heel ask the client to raise the heel off the support. If the knee raises first before heel is raised then quadriceps lag is present.

4. *Dynamic tibial rotatory function (Helfet test):* In high sitting position mark the tibial tubercle and midline of patella by a skin marker and note their relationship with other. Normally, tibial tubercle lines up with the midline or lateral half of patella. As the knee extends tibia rotates through 10–15° over the final 20–30° of extension. Loss of dynamic tibial rotation may be secondary to tight or adherent medial capsule-ligamentous structures

or internal derangement such as meniscus displacement or cartilaginous loose body.

5. *Rotation of tibia on femur:* In high sitting position with the knee flexed to 90° ask the client to rotate the leg medially and laterally and note the range, pain. Normally, range of medial rotation is 30° and lateral rotation 40°.

6. *Passive movements:* Knee flexion-extension in supine position and record the range of motion, end-feel, crepitus, pain, etc. Check medial rotation and lateral rotation range of motion, end-feel and pain with the knee flexed to 90°. Pain during lateral rotation of tibia could be due to sprain MCL or medial meniscus.

7. Passive hip movements to test length of hamstrings, rectus femoris, iliotibial band (ITB), hip flexors, external rotators and adductors. For hamstrings check the straight-leg raise (SLR) with the pelvis fixed in supine position or fix the thigh with hip flexed to 90° and then straighten the knee, measure the range deficient from 0° of knee extension.

Prone knee bending test for rectus femoris, in prone position on passive flexion of knee, client's same side hip will spontaneously flex indicating tightness of rectus femoris on that side.

Ober's test for tensor fascia lata (TFL) and iliotibial (IT) band, in side lying position on the sound side with underlying hip and knee flexed for stability, passively fix the pelvis by one hand and with the other hand passively abduct, extend and adduct the hip with the knee flexed to 90°. The involved thigh will not fall to the bed indicating tightness of TFL and ITB. In case of iliotibial band tightness full passive knee extension will not be possible from the above position.

Hip external rotators tightness can be tested bilaterally in prone with the knees flexed to 90° and checking internal rotation range on both the sides.

Thomas test for hip flexors, in supine position passively flex the sound hip and knee till increased lumbar lordosis is obliterated, if the opposite thigh is raised off the bed then the test is positive indicating hip flexor tightness. If flexion of sound side hip and knee does not obliterate increased lumbar lordosis, flex both hip and knees then gradually extend affected hip. Limitation of hip extension indicate hip flexor tightness, limitation of hip internal rotation indicate iliopsoas tightness, limitation of knee flexion indicate rectus femoris tightness, limitation of hip adduction suggest ITB/TFL tightness.

Hip adductors tightness can be detected by checking abduction range in crook lying position. Limitation of hip abduction range more with the knee straight than that with knee flexed indicate long adductors tightness.

8. Joint play:
   - Anterior to posterior gliding of tibia on femur
   - Posterior to anterior gliding of tibia on femur
   - Medial rotation of tibia on femur
   - Lateral rotation of tibia on femur
   - Cephalocaudal gliding and caudalo-cephal gliding of patella
   - Medial to lateral and lateral to medial gliding of patella
   - Anterior to posterior and posterior to anterior glide of fibular head.
9. Resisted isometric contraction:
   - Knee flexion—hamstrings
   - Knee extension—quadriceps
   - Lateral rotation of tibia on femur—biceps femoris
   - Medial rotation of tibia on femur—pes anserinus tendons.

IV. Neuromuscular Evaluation

1. Sensation of lower extremity
2. *Deep tendon reflexes (DTR):* Knee jerk (L3, 4), medial hamstrings (L5), ankle jerk (S1, 2)
3. Manual muscle testing—hip flexors (L2), quadriceps (L3), tibialis anterior (L4), toe extensors/tibialis posterior (L5), plantar flexors (S1, 2), hip extensors (S1), knee flexors (S1, 2)
4. Bowel and bladder functions.

V. Palpation

1. *Patella:* size, shape and position, a small high ridding patella is susceptible to subluxation/dislocation. Tenderness over inferior pole patella is the common site for jumper's knee. Passively push the patella medially to palpate its medial facet, which becomes tender in lateral tracking dysfunction. With the knee in extension fat pad is normally extruded to the either side of patellar tendon, which become tender in case of fat pad syndrome.

2. *Femoral condyles:* Palpate the anterior projection of lateral femoral condyle, adductor tubercle.
3. *Proximal tibia:* Palpate the insertion of pes anserinus tendons, medial collateral ligament, ITB, fibular head and tibial tubercle.

Skin

Temperature, texture, tenderness, moisture and mobility.

Smooth, warm, glossy and wet skin indicate hypervascularity and is the characteristic feature of acute inflammation or acute reflex sympathetic dystrophy; whereas rough, dry, scaly, cold skin indicate hypovascularity and is characteristic feature of chronic inflammation or chronic reflex sympathetic dystrophy.

Fluctuation test: Place one hand over the suprapatellar pouch and other hand below the inferior pole of patella. By pressing down with one hand impulse of the dispersed fluid will be felt by the other hand indicating significant effusion.

Patellar tap test: Milking the fluid distally out of the suprapatellar pouch with one hand, tap over the patella by other lateral three fingers tips. Floating of the patella will be felt indicating significant effusion.

Palpate the muscles, tendons and ligaments for their continuity, consistency and mobility. For MCL palpate the medial tibiofemoral joint line and move the finger backward until the gap is no more palpable by the presence of MCL. Lateral collateral ligament (LCL) can be easily palpable in figure four sitting position, between the head of fibula and femur.

Peripheral pulsations: Femoral, popliteal, posterior tibial and dorsalis pedis arteries for rate, rhythm, volume, bilateral synchronous, proximal and distal deficit, etc.

VI. Special Tests

1. **Valgus stress test (Fig. 2.1)** is done to assess medial instability (one plane).
   - *Position of subject*: Supine lying
   - *Position of the therapist*: Stands by the supporting the knee in 30° of flexion by one hand and the ankle with the other hand,

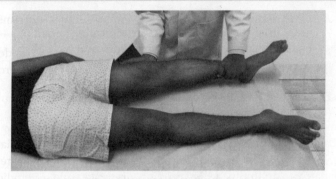

Fig. 2.1: Valgus stress test.

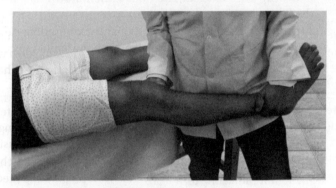

Fig. 2.2: Varus stress test.

pushes the knee medially to apply valgus stress while the ankle
is stabilized.

- *Response:* The test is said to be positive when tibia moves
away from the femur excessively indicating sprain of medial
collateral ligament. If the test becomes positive with the knee
in extension then MCL, posteromedial joint capsule and ACL
are injured.

2. **Varus stress test (Fig. 2.2)** is done to assess lateral instability (one
plane).
    - Position of subject: Supine lying.
    - *Position of the therapist:* Stands by the supporting the knee in
    30° of flexion by one hand and the ankle with the other hand,
    pushes the knee laterally to apply varus stress while the ankle
    is stabilized.

- *Response*: The test is said to be positive when tibia moves away from the femur excessively indicating sprain of lateral collateral ligament. If the test becomes positive with the knee in extension then LCL, posterolateral joint capsule and PCL are injured.

3. **Drawer test (Fig. 2.3)** is done to assess anteroposterior instability (one plane).
   - *Position of subject*: Crook lying with hip flexed to 45°, knee 90° and foot flat on the bed.
   - *Position of the therapist*: Sitting over patient's forefoot to fix the foot and places the hands around the upper tibia to ensure hamstrings are relaxed. The tibia is then drawn forward on the femur.
   - *Response*: The test is said to be positive when tibia moves forward excessively (more than 6 mm) on the femur indicating sprain ACL.

4. **Sag sign:**
   - *Position of subject*: Crook lying with hips flexed to 45°, knees 90° and feet flat on the bed.
   - *Position of the therapist*: Observes the tibial tubercle from the side.
   - *Response:* In this position, the tibia drops back or sags back on the femur indicating torn PCL.

5. **Godfrey's chair test (Fig. 2.4):**
   - *Position of subject*: Crook lying with hips and knees flexed to 70–80°, heels supported on seat of a chair.
   - *Position of the therapist*: Observes the tibial tubercle from the side.

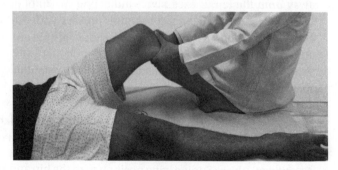

Fig. 2.3: Drawer test.

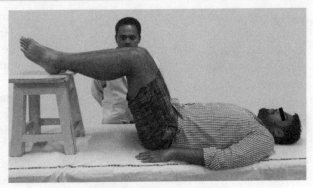

Fig. 2.4: Godfrey's chair test.

- *Response:* In this position, the tibia drops back or displaces back on the femur indicating torn PCL.

6. **Active posterior drawer test:**
   - *Position of subject:* Crook lying with hips flexed to 45°, knees 90° and feet flat on the bed. With the foot fixed on the bed client is asked to contract quadriceps and try to extend the knee by pushing the foot down towards the bed end.
   - *Response*: Normally, the tibial remains in neutral or moves slightly posteriorly. In case of this torn PCL, the tibia will move forward because of the unbalanced force vectors of quadriceps and patellar tendon.

7. **Lachman test (Fig. 2.5)** is done for ACL when the knee can only be flexed to 15–20°.
   - *Position of subject*: Semisitting position with the back supported.
   - *Position of the therapist*: Client's ankle is stabilized between Therapist's legs. Move the proximal tibia forward with the hands.
   - Alternately in supine position therapist's one hand stabilizes the thigh and with the other hand moves the proximal tibia forward.
   - *Response*: The degree of anterior translation and firmness are noted. Lachman test of soft end-feel is diagnostic of ACL tear. 1+ = 5 mm, 2+ = 10 mm, 3+ = 15 mm, 4+ = 20 mm.

8. **McMurray test (Fig. 2.6):**
   - *Position of subject*: Supine lying position with the hip and knee flexed to 90°.

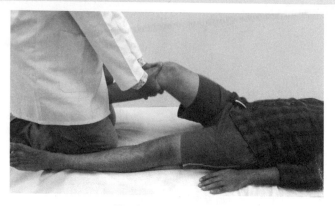

Fig. 2.5: Lachman test.

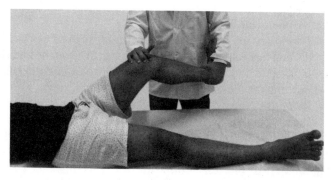

Fig. 2.6: McMurray test.

- *Position of the therapist*: Support the knee with one hand and grasp above the ankle, rotate the leg laterally and extend it.
- *Response:* Pain or click during the maneuver indicates tear of anterior horn of the medial meniscus.

In supine lying position with the knee fully flexed, rotate the leg laterally and extend the knee to 90°. Pain or click during the maneuver indicates tear of posterior horn of the medial meniscus. The test may be modified by medially rotating the leg and extending the knee for lateral meniscus.

9. **Apley's test (Fig. 2.7):**
   - *Position of subject:* Prone lying position with the knee flexed to 90°.

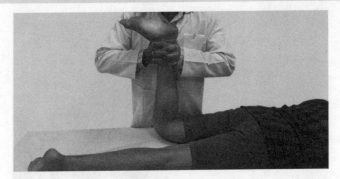

Fig. 2.7: Apley's test.

- *Position of the therapist:* Client's thigh is fixed to the bed by Therapist's knee. Medially and laterally rotate the leg combined with distraction. Repeat medial and lateral rotation combined with compression. Note restriction and pain.
- *Response:*
  - Medial rotation and distraction—cruciates
  - Lateral rotation and distraction—collateral ligament
  - Medial rotation and compression—lateral meniscus
  - Lateral rotation and compression—medial meniscus.

10. **Steinmann's sign:** Steinmann's sign is useful in the presence of anterior joint line tenderness. Pain appears to move anteriorly with knee extension and posteriorly with flexion indicates meniscus tear. Rotation of the leg with the knee flexed to 90° may localize the pain at the joint.

11. **Jerk test of Hughston (Fig. 2.8):**
    - *Position of subject:* Supine lying with hip flexed to 45° and knee 90°.
    - *Position of the therapist:* With one hand supports the knee and other hand grasps above the ankle, internally rotate the leg and apply valgus stress to the knee, gradually straighten the knee.
    - *Response:* At about 30° of extension, the lateral tibial condyle may sublax or jerks forward suddenly. As the knee further extends, the tibia returns to its former position indicating anterolateral instability.

12. **Pivot shift test of MacIntosh (Fig. 2.9):** This is the primary test used to assess anterolateral rotary instability of the knee.
    - *Position of subject:* Supine lying with hip flexed to 20° and knee slightly flexed 5°.

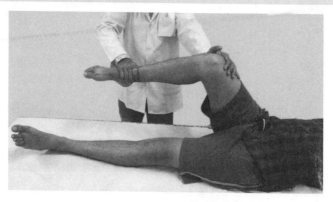

Fig. 2.8: Jerk test of Hughston.

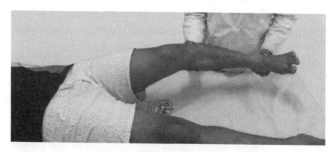

Fig. 2.9: Pivot shift test of MacIntosh.

– *Position of the therapist:* With one hand supports the knee and other hand grasps above the ankle, internally rotate the leg and apply valgus stress to the knee, gradually flexes the knee.
– *Response:* At about 30° of flexion, the tibia will reduce or jerk backward. The client will say that is what the giving way feels like indicating injury of posterolateral capsule, LCL and ACL.

13. **Hughston's posterolateral and posteromedial drawer sign (Figs. 2.10A and B):**
    – *Position of subject:* Supine lying with hip flexed to 45°, knee 90° and foot flat on the bed.
    – *Position of the therapist:* Medially rotate the leg and sit over the forefoot to stabilize it. Push the tibia posteriorly.
    – *Response:* If the tibia moves or rotates posteriorly on the medial aspect excessively as compared to the sound side, the test is

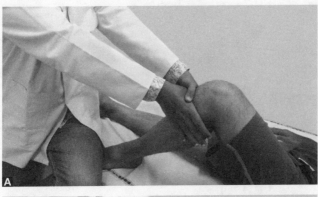

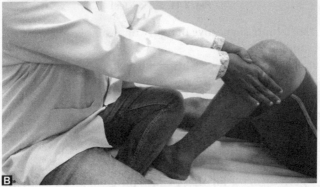

Figs. 2.10A and B: (A) Hughston's posterolateral test; (B) Posteromedial test.

positive indicative of posteromedial instability suggestive of injury posteromedial capsule, MCL, PCL.

Posterolateral instability may be tested similarly with the leg rotated laterally. Excessive posterior rotation of tibia on its lateral aspect as compared to the sound side indicates injury of posterolateral capsule, LCL and PCL.

14. **Slocum test (Fig. 2.11):**
    - *Position of subject:* Supine lying with hip flexed to 45° and knee 90° and foot flat on the bed.
    - *Position of the therapist:* Medially rotate the leg and sit over the forefoot to stabilize it. Draw the tibia forward.
    - *Response:* If the movement on the lateral aspect is more than that on the sound side indicative of anterolateral rotary

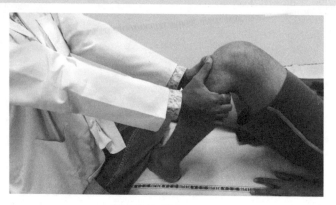

Fig. 2.11: Slocum test.

instability suggestive of injury of posterolateral capsule, ACL and LCL.

For anteromedial rotary instability, rotate the tibia laterally and draw the tibia forward. Excessive forward movement of the medial aspect more than that on the sound side indicative of anteromedial rotatory instability suggestive of injury of posteromedial capsule, MCL and ACL.

15. **External rotation and recurvatum test (Fig. 2.12):**
    – *Position of subject:* Supine lying with the knees straight.
    – *Position of the therapist:* Grasp the great toes of both the feet.
    – *Response:* Knee with posterolateral instability will go into hyperextension at the lateral side, tibia will externally rotate and medial aspect of the knee will show an apparent tibia vara.

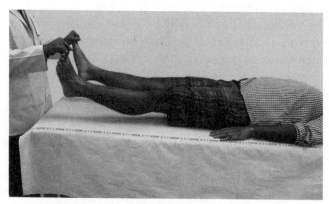

Fig. 2.12: External rotation and recurvatum test.

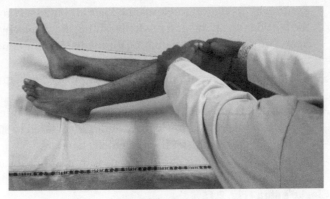

Fig. 2.13: Plica test.

16. **Plica test (Fig. 2.13):** A pathological process affecting the synovial plica can mimic a meniscal injury and cause symptoms that are not unlike those of other common internal derangements of the knee; this makes differential diagnosis more difficult. A symptomatic mediopatellar plica can often be palpated as a tender, band-like structure paralleling the medial border of the patella. A palpable and sometimes audible snap is present during flexion and extension.
    – *Position of subject*: Supine lying with knee flexed to 30°.
    – *Position of the therapist*: Move the patella medially.
    – *Response*: Pain caused by the edge of plica being pinched between medial femoral condyle and patella.

17. **Hughston plica test (Fig. 2.14):**
    – *Position of subject*: Supine lying position.

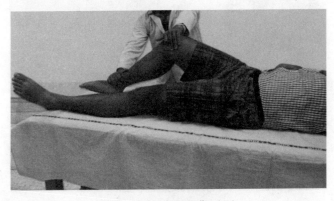

Fig. 2.14: Hughston plica test.

- *Position of the therapist*: Flexes the knee and medially rotate the leg with one hand and medially gliding the patella by the heel of other hand while palpating the medial femoral condyle with the fingers.
- *Response*: A tender popping of the plica fold may be palpated indicating a positive test.

18. **Apprehension test:** Patellar stability can be judged by this test.
    - *Position of subject:* Supine lying with the knee flexed to 30°.
    - *Position of the therapist:* Push the patella laterally.
    - *Response:* Contraction of quadriceps to prevent dislocation and apprehension look of the client indicate the test is positive.

19. **Clarke's sign (Fig. 2.15):**
    - *Position of subject:* Supine lying position.
    - *Position of the therapist:* Push the patella caudally by the web of the hand and the client is asked to contract his quadriceps.
    - *Response:* Retropatellar pain and inability to hold the contraction indicates the test is positive suggestive of chondromalacia patella.

20. **Arnold's test:**[2]
    - *Position of subject:* Single leg standing on the involved site. Ask the patient to rotate his upright torso of face about 90° in opposite direction by crossing his good leg over the fix one.
    - *Response:* Feeling of discomfort, lateral pivot shift and the sensation of knee wanting to go out indicate instability.

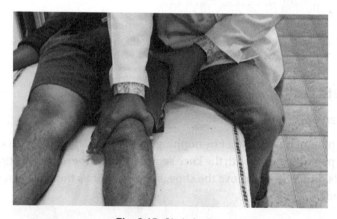

Fig. 2.15: Clarke's sign.

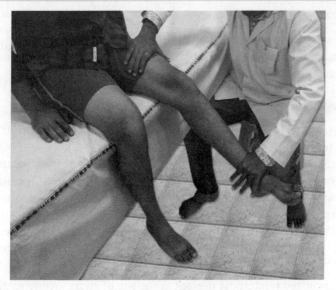

Fig. 2.16: McConnell test.

21. **McConnell test (Fig. 2.16):**[3]
   - *Position of the subject*: High sitting with femur laterally rotated. Ask the patient to isometrically contracts the quadriceps muscle for 10 seconds in various angle of knee flexion (0, 30°,60°, 90°, 120°).
   - If the pain is produced, test is repeated with the therapist holding a medial glide to the patella, if the symptoms are ease indicates chondromalacia patella.

Acute Lesion with Effusion

Observation

The patient reports either by hopping or carried by the care-givers or by a pair of crutches with the knee semiflexed and toe touch position. Finds difficulty to remove the shoe, sock, trouser as the knee can be flexed.

Inspection

Knee assumes semiflexed position to accommodate the effusion. Suprapatellar girth measurement is increased. Overlying skin becomes red, shiny and glossy.

Movements

1. Active weight-bearing movement is not possible.
2. Active non-weight-bearing knee flexion-extension is restricted in capsular pattern.
3. Passive movements are restricted in capsular pattern with muscle spasm end-feel. Joint play cannot be assessed properly due to spasm.
4. Resisted isometric contraction should be strong and painless.

Palpation

1. Localized tenderness present at the site of injury, overlying skin becomes warm, moist.
2. Fluctuation test and patellar tap test are positive. Hemarthrosis may accompany cruciate tear, meniscus tear, intra-articular fracture.

Special tests

Special tests to be done to clinically diagnose the ligamentous injury.

Acute Lesion without Effusion

Absence of effusion following recent injury indicates either the injury is mild or there is complete rupture of the capsuloligamentous structures, so that the effusion tracks out of the joint cavity through the rupture site. In the absence of effusion the knee can be straighten and good range of knee movements will be present. There will be no pain since no intact nerve ending is left. Later on as muscle spasm develops to guard the joint instability some pain may be experienced, which is not proportional to the severity of injury. In the absence of effusion, pain and deformity the patient may be able to walk without aids.

Observation

The patient reports walking without any walking aids.

Inspection

Knee is almost straight.

Movements

1. Active weight-bearing movement may not be possible.
2. Active non-weight-bearing and passive knee flexion-extension is almost full. Joint play demonstrates hypermobility due to ligamentous instability.
3. Resisted isometric contraction should be strong and painless.

Palpation

Localized tenderness present at the site of injury.

Special Tests

Special tests to be done to clinically diagnose the ligamentous injury.

Chronic Lesion without Effusion

Patient with chronic ligamentous injury complains of functional instability or giving way of the knee during particular activity. Inability to turn quickly in case of collateral ligament, inability to run forward in case of ACL and inability to squat, descend stairs, running with sudden stop, running backward, etc. in case of PCL injury.

Quadriceps atrophy is one of the significant findings. Active and passive joint range of motion is good. Joint play demonstrates ligamentous instability and special test is diagnostic.

REFERENCES

1. Brotzman S, et al. Clinical orthopaedic rehabilitation. 2nd edition: p. 253.
2. Joshi J, et al. Essentials of orthopaedics and applied physiotherapy, 2nd edition; 2010.p.547.
3. Petty N. Neuromusculoskeletal examination and assessment: a hand book for therapist, 2nd edition.p. 327.

Chapter **3**

Soft Tissue Injuries

Knee joint pathologies are commonly of traumatic origin. Knee is freely movable in sagittal plane. Thus, forces acting to move the knee in frontal and transverse planes are largely attenuated as internal strain to soft tissues about the joint. Furthermore such force may act over the relatively long lever arms provided by femurs and tibia thereby increasing the potential loading of the structures. Therefore, soft tissue injuries about the knee joint are very common.

MEDIAL COLLATERAL LIGAMENT INJURY

Medial collateral ligament (MCL) is long and flat, attached to medial epicondyle to medial aspect of shaft of tibia about 4 cm below the joint line. It lies slightly anterior to the joint axis. It becomes taut in extension, abduction and external rotation of tibia and some of the anterior fibers become taut in flexion. It also prevents anterior displacement of tibia on femur. Its deep capsular fibers are attached to medial meniscus and compromises its mobility. Anteromedially medial patellar retinaculum and posteromedially pes anserinus tendons (Gracilis, semitendinosus, and sartorius) and semimembranosus prevent excessive abduction, external rotation and anterior displacement of tibia. They reinforce the medial collateral ligament.

Functional Anatomy

The MCL is the major stabilizing structure for the medial aspect of the knee joint protecting the knee from valgus (lateral to medial) forces. The MCL is divided into deep MCL (d-MCL), superficial MCL (s-MCL) and posterior oblique ligament, these are called static stabilizer of the medial knee. Dynamic stabilizer include musculotendinous unit of semimembranosus, quadriceps and pes anserinus. A bursae separates the superficial and deep MCL, which is a small jelly filled sac that reduces friction between the two segments, so it allows anteroposterior excursion of the s-MCL during flexion and extension. The superficial portion of the ligament is broad that arises proximally from the medial epicondyle on the femur and attaches 4–5 cm distal to the joint line on the medial surface of the tibia posterior to pes anserinus. Its anterior fibers become taut during flexion and lax during full extension. The deep portion lies just beneath the superficial portion and has a firm attachment to the medial meniscus and the fibrous capsule surrounding the knee joint (Moore, 1996). Posterior to the MCL is the posteromedial corner, made of the capsule called the posterior oblique ligament (POL). This complex is tight in extension and become confluent with the posterior joint capsule.[1-3] The MCL is primary restraint against valgus stress. At 25° of flexion, MCL provides 78% of the valgus-restraining force. In extension, the ACL, POL, medial meniscus, semimembranosus also contribute to valgus stress and MCL provides 57% of the restraining force against valgus stress. In general, an isolated MCL tear lead to valgus laxity in flexion, while additional injury to the secondary restraint (ACL) leads to increase laxity in extension.[1-3]

Gardiner et al. found that the amount of strain to valgus stress over different areas depends on flexion angle of knee.

1. In full knee extension, strain occurs over the posterior part of MCL.
2. Throughout different flexion angle—strain remains constant on anterior fibers.
3. Several radiographic studies confirm that posterofemoral attachment is common site of injury.

With valgus stress, there is tension over the medial aspect of the knee joint leading to stretching of MCL. A minor MCL sprain is a common lesion that usually occurs from an external rotation strain of tibia on the femur. Depending on the amount of force, there will be variable degrees of MCL sprain. One of the most common mechanisms occur when a football player is tackled from the side with the foot planted and the knee slightly flexed. The victim is usually struck while trying to turn or cut away. The forces on the knee include a valgus stress, external rotation of the tibia on the femur and usually an anterior movement of the tibia on the femur (Fig. 3.1).

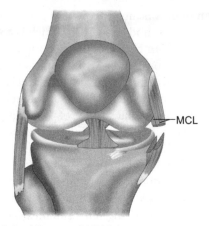

Fig. 3.1: Medial collateral ligament (MCL) injury.

(*Source:* Injuries to the medial collateral ligament of the knee. 2013.https://phoenixshoulderandknee.com/).

With severe sprain, there will be damage to medial joint capsule. If the force becomes more, there will be injury to medial meniscus to which the deep fibers of MCL gets attached. If the force further exceeds, there will be injury to anterior cruciate ligament (ACL). The conditions in which all these three ligaments are damaged are known as triad of O'Donoghue. Similar type of injury on the medial aspect of the knee joint is uncommon as both the medial sides are well protected.

Grade I (mild) sprain is essentially a stretch injury. Only a few fibers are disrupted. Valgus opening: 0–5 mm.[1] Anatomical and functional integrity of the structure are maintained. Anatomical integrity is checked by valgus stress test, which is characterized by pain but no increase in amplitude of abduction of tibia over femur. Functional integrity is determined by the level of activities and disability. Patient may complaint of pain during running and turning away from the affected side but no giving way. Localized tenderness present.

Grade II (Moderate) sprain is partial tear of the capsule-ligamentous structures. Damage of more fibers but some fibers are still intact. Valgus opening: 5-10 mm.[1] Generalized tenderness. There is loss of anatomical as well as functional integrity of the structure. Instability can be demonstrated by valgus stress test which shows hyperabduction of tibia over femur with pain. Functionally pain and

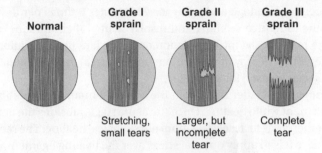

Grade I sprain — Stretching, small tears
Grade II sprain — Larger, but incomplete tear
Grade III sprain — Complete tear
Normal

Fig. 3.2: Grades of ligament sprain.
(*Source:* Sprain or Strain – What is the Difference. Kintec. 2016. http://www.kintec.net).

giving way present during running and turning away from the affected side. Associated involvement of capsular ligament gives rise to joint effusion with limitation of range of motion in capsular pattern.

Grade-III (severe) sprain is complete rupture of the capsule-ligamentous structures. All ligamentous structures are damaged giving rise to complete loss of anatomical as well as functional integrity of the structure. Valgus opening : >10 mm.[1] Instability can be demonstrated by valgus stress test which shows hyperabduction of tibia over femur without pain. Functionally, there will be giving way during running and turning away from the affected side. No effusion or limitation movement present (Fig. 3.2).

Lateral collateral ligament is short and rounded, attached to the lateral epicondyle of femur to the head of fibula. It does not get attached to the lateral meniscus. Popliteus tendon runs underneath it, i.e. between lateral meniscus and LCL. It is covered by the biceps femoris tendon. It lies slightly posterior to the joint axis. It becomes taut in extension, adduction and external rotation of tibia.

Conservative Management

Medial collateral ligament sprain grade I is unimportant and persons with grade I sprain usually manage it by self-treatment. Measures to relief the pain only have to be taken.

Medial collateral ligament sprain sprain grade II is important for physiotherapy point of view. During the acute stage, the aim of physiotherapy is to prevent further damage, early resolution of the inflammation and pain relief. Keep the part in elevation with compressive bandage and apply ice 20 minutes 5 times per day for 48 hours to reduce swelling and resolve acute inflammation. High voltage pulsed galvanic stimulation or strong faradic stimulation or interferential therapy or transcutaneous electrical nerve stimulation (TENS) can be used for pain relief.

Immediately after the sprain the aim is to maintain mobility of the ligament while healing. Once the acute stage subsides the aim of physiotherapy is to accelerate more physiological healing. The means to achieve it is to apply optimal stress over the healing ligament.

Cyriax's deep transverse friction massage can be applied at the joint line, where it is attached to the medial meniscus, across the ligament in different positions of knee flexion-extension to prevent/breaks the adhesion of healing ligament and increases the extensibility, restore mobility and to realign the newly produced collagen perpendicular to the direction of stress. Care must be taken not to apply at the proximal attachment of MCL, which may give rise to periosteal disruption and heterotrophic bone formation. It also disperses inflammatory exudates relieving pain and preventing adhesion.

The patient lies on the couch and therapist's index finger reinforced by the middle finger lies over the affected part of the ligament and thumb on the outer side of the joint. By alternately flexing and extending the wrist, the fingers move to and fro over the ligament with adequate pressure and sweep, keeping the thumb still as the fulcrum fixed. Thus, the ligament moves over the underlying bone. As the initial pain and discomfort disappears gradually increase the pressure and again as the pain and discomfort disappears gradually increase the pressure further. The frequency of movement is 2/second. The treatment is applied for about 10 minutes followed by active movements and passive stretching.

Alternately optimal stress over the healing ligament can be applied by applying valgus stress in supine position with the knee in about 10° of flexion or external rotation of tibia in prone with the knee in 90° of flexion.

Mulligan's mobilization with movements: Patient in prone lying and therapist stands on the contralateral side. The belt is placed around the waist and patient's lower leg so that the proximal edge is at the tibial joint margin. The thigh is stabilized above the knee by one hand and the leg is supported by the other hand. Glide the tibia medially with the belt while the patient flexes and extends the knee painlessly.

Therapist in sitting position, patient stands in the front placing his foot of the affected side on the chair in-between therapist's knee. Therapist places his thumb reinforced by the other thumb over the joint line on the MCL. With the thumb pressure maintained, ask the subject to alternately flex and extend the knee.

Passive, active-assisted range of motion (ROM) exercise within pain free range are given after a few days. ROM exercise in cold whirl pool bath can be given immediately followed by warm whirl pool bath after a few days. Static quadriceps, straight leg raise (SLR) can be initiated from the next day and as the acuteness subsides active knee flexion, cycling, swimming, SLR in all directions except hip adduction, etc. can be added.

2nd week progressive resisted knee extension, multiangle quadriceps exercise, hamstrings curls, hip adduction, closed kinetic exercise and stretching of hamstrings, quadriceps, TA, iliotibial band (ITB) are given. Full weight-bearing is allowed once full range without any pain and swelling is achieved followed by balance training.

Grade III isolated MCL rupture can be managed non-surgically as MCL has an excellent secondary support system, weight-bearing force tends to compress the medial aspect aiding the stability. The injury can be protected adequately in hinged brace to avoid valgus stress, prevent atrophy. Nonweight-bearing exercises are performed for weeks and partial weight-bearing for 3 months with the functional knee brace. Progressive strengthening, endurance, stretching exercises are given. After 3 months balance exercises and gradual running can be added.

Giannotti et al.[4,5] published guidelines for a functional rehabilitation program after isolated grade 3 MCL injuries. They state that "good to excellent results can be expected with a return to full preinjury activity level being the norm." A simple hinged knee brace is used initially to protect the knee from valgus stress. Depending on the activity, bracing may be continued until the patient feels stable and safe playing without it. The protocol outlines four phases covering a time span of 10–12 weeks. During phase 1 (0–4 weeks), goals are to decrease swelling, restore knee range of motion from 0–100°, gain 4/5 quadriceps and hamstring strength, restore a normal gait pattern, and restore full-weight-bearing status. Treatment during phase 1 includes cryotherapy, electrical muscle stimulation, stretching, range of motion exercises, and quadriceps and hamstring strengthening. During phase 2 (4–6 weeks), goals are to continue to control swelling, restore full knee range of motion from 0–140°, and gain 5/5 quadriceps and hamstring strength. Treatment during phase 2 includes cryotherapy, closed chain exercises, and static proprioceptive exercises. During phase 3 (6–10 weeks) goals are to regain the ability to perform squats, return to light jogging and agility skills, and possibly progress to sport-specific skills and competition. Treatment during phase 3 includes treadmill jogging, dynamic proprioceptive exercises, slide board training and rebounder training. During phase 4 (8–12 weeks) goals are to attain 95% quadriceps index and 90% single leg hop index, return to full running and sport-specific drills, and resume competition. Treatment during phase 4 includes plyometric training, full agility and sport-specific drills, continued dynamic proprioceptive exercises and rebounder training, and road running. In general, return to competition is allowed after the following are achieved: there are no signs or symptoms of instability and there is a normal ligament exam; quadriceps strength is at least 90% when compared to the contralateral extremity; and sport-specific skills, agility testing, and athletic activities do not cause any pain.

Repair/Reconstruction

Immobilization in plaster cylinder or hinged cast brace is given for 3–6 weeks, during which static quadriceps, hamstrings exercises, SLR and ankle foot exercises should be done. Patellar mobilization, and electrical stimulation (ES) to quadriceps can be given.

After plaster removal, US followed by deep transverse friction massage (DTFM) are given over the ligament to improve its mobility. Then controlled mobilization technique followed by active movement is encouraged. Partial weight-bearing in hinged cast brace is allowed once about 10° knee extension is achieved.

After 6 weeks progressive strengthening, endurance, stretching and passive mobilization should be given.

Once full extension with adequate strength is achieved balance training is given, then patient returns back to activity.

Early Mobilization Protocol

2 weeks: Active ankle foot and toe movements, static quadriceps exercise, SLR, passive ROM exercise by lying in prone for knee extension, wall sliding once 80–90° range is achieved, patellar mobilization, ES are given.

Partial weight-bearing crutch walking with the brace locked in extension can be initiated once full knee extension is achieved.

2–4 weeks: 120° ROM should be regained by 4th week, active knee flexion followed by resisted, resisted SLR, cycling, closed kinetic chain (CKC) exercise, balance training, active knee extension 90–60°, Full weight-bearing can be allowed by 3–4 weeks.

4–6 week: Full joint range of motion (FJROM) should be regained by 6th week, 90–40° active knee extension.

8–10 week: Activity

12 weeks: FJROM, full knee extension and adequate strength

16–18 weeks: Jogging can be initiated once quadriceps become 65% of the sound side.

5–6 months: Return to sports once quadriceps become 80% of the sound side.

MENISCUS INJURY

Anatomy

Medial and lateral menisci are semicircular fibrocartilaginous structure that deepens the tibial articulating surfaces. Their anterior horns are attached in front of the intercondylar area of tibia and posterior horns behind it. Medial meniscus is semicircular in shape, forms part of a larger circle whereas lateral meniscus forms almost of a smaller circle as its both the horns are attached close to each other. Peripherally joint capsule is attached to the upper margin of the menisci and coronary ligament, which constitutes the inferior aspect of the joint capsule, is attached to the lower margin of the menisci. MCL is attached to the medial meniscus but LCL is not attached to the lateral meniscus. Therefore, lateral meniscus is more mobile, whereas medial meniscus is less mobile owing to its extensive peripheral attachment. Medial meniscus translates 2–5 mm whereas lateral meniscus translates 9–11 mm in the anteroposterior plane. That is the reason why medial meniscus is more prone to injury.

Peripheral one-third of menisci are vascular, supplied by branches from the superior, inferior and lateral geniculate arteries. The middle-third is not completely avascular as it receives some blood supply, whereas inner-third is avascular, is nourished by synovial fluid diffusion.

Menisci are one of the protectors of knee. It provides congruity to the articulating surfaces; absorb shock and reduces the stress. Forces across the knee joint may be as high as 2–4 times body weight during walking and up to 6–8 times body weight during running. Menisci transmit approximately 50% of the load and about 90% of load at 90° of knee flexion. The lateral meniscus transmits greater percentage of load in the lateral compartment (approximately 70%) where as medial meniscus transmits approximately 50% of load in the medial compartment. Surgical excision of meniscus can result in alteration in knee joint function, degeneration of articular cartilage, reduction in joint space, osteophyte formation, alteration in shape of femoral condyle, etc. It also helps in lubrication and nutrition to the joint. During loading of the knee, when the meniscus is compressed, synovial fluid is driven into the articular cartilage.

Menisci move with the tibia in flexion-extension and with femur in rotation. Normally, external rotation of tibia in nonweight-bearing or internal rotation of femur in weight-bearing occurs during terminal knee extension and internal rotation of tibia in nonweight-bearing or external rotation of femur in weight-bearing occurs during initial flexion. Full extension is possible in the absence of normal rotation, but at the expense of deformation of articular tissues, i.e. sprain meniscus. Flexion-extension without rotation or with abnormal rotation put stress over the meniscus giving rise to injury. Rotation at complete extension is not possible, but forced rotation put stress over the meniscus. In extension, the menisci are at their extreme forward position, with rotation either of the menisci tends to move forward and the other tends to move back. There will be excessive stress over the former leading to injury. Similarly in hyperflexed knee, i.e. in squatting, where the menisci are at their extreme posterior position, rotation in either direction will tend to move one of the menisci backward and the other forward. The one which tends to move back will have excessive stress; it cannot move further backward and gets injured.

Epidemiology

The mean annual incidence of meniscal lesions has been reported to be 66 per 100,000 inhabitants, 61 of which result in meniscectomy (Makris et al. 2011). A meniscus tear (Fig. 3.3) can be located in any location, and in any conceivable pattern. Anterior horn tears are unusual. Tears typically begin in the posterior horn and progress anteriorly. Patients with sports injuries are usually in mid-thirty years, and account for approximately 33% of cases. Patients with non-sporting injuries are in fourth decade of life, and account for approximately 39% of cases. Patients with an indefinable injury have a mean age of 43 years, and account for about 29% of cases. There is a 4:1 male to female ratio in these tears, and approximately 2/3 of all cases occur in the medial meniscus. It should also be noted that associated ACL tears were found in 47% of the patients in sports injuries and in 13% of the non-sporting injuries. In the no-injury group, there were no ACL tears. In chronic ACL injuries medial meniscus tear occurrence is 36%, lateral meniscus tear occurrence is 22% and both menisci tear occurrence is 16%.[6-9]

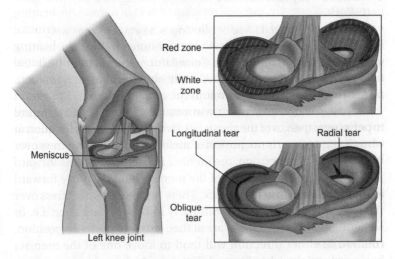

Fig. 3.3: Meniscus tear.

(*Source:* Miller J. Meniscus tear. http://physioworks.com.au/).

Clinical Features

The onset is usually sudden with an immediate deep pain associated with giving way of the joint. If hemarthrosis occurs, there will be severe diffuse pain and tense swelling arising within minutes of injury. In the absence of severe effusion pain is localized at the site of injury on the joint line. Longitudinal tear of medial meniscus extending anteriorly often gets displaced interfering with the normal joint mechanics resulting in locking of the joint so that terminal 20–30 of extension will be lost. Locking is usually preceded by previous minor incidences of giving way followed by effusion.

The severity of symptoms can vary for different types of meniscal tears. The most common meniscal tear pattern is a single longitudinal tear, which is traumatic in origin. A long central fragment attached at each to the meniscal horns progressed over time to become bucket handle tear. When the unstable bucket handle fragment displaces into the intercondylar notch, it blocks full extension of knee and quite painful. Horizontal/transverse tears often results of chronic degenerative changes and usually occurs in elderly. It may progress to become flap tear. Radial tears occur in the central aspect of the meniscus, which progress peripherally to become parrot beak tear. Transverse or radial tear move in and out of the joint without locking the joint, but may cause occasional symptoms of giving way, mild pain and effusion.

Patient with locked knee or effusion is hesitant to bear weight. As the effusion subsides and movement is restored patient can resume activities with little or no pain. Complaint of intermittent buckling or locking followed by effusion. Altered joint mechanics gives rise to persistent clicks and there develops quadriceps wasting.

Vascularity of menisci decrease from periphery to central. Injury to peripheral margin of meniscus has favorable prognosis for healing whereas injury to central portion of meniscus has poor prognosis for healing.

Physical Examination

Acute Stage

Observation

The patient reports either by hopping or carried by the care-givers or by a pair of crutches with the knee semiflexed and toe touch position.

Finds difficulty to remove the shoe, sock, trouser as the knee can be flexed.

Inspection
Knee assumes semiflexed position to accommodate the effusion. Suprapatellar girth measurement is increased. Overlying skin becomes red, shiny and glossy.

Movements
1. Active weight-bearing movement is not possible.
2. Active nonweight-bearing knee flexion-extension is restricted in capsular pattern. Considerable loss of extension is present if the knee is locked.
3. Passive movements are restricted in capsular pattern with muscle spasm end-feel and springy rebound end feel in case of locked knee.
4. Joint play cannot be assessed properly due to spasm. External rotation of tibia is painful in case of medial meniscus injury.
5. Resisted isometric contraction should be strong and painless.

Palpation
1. Localized tenderness present at the site of injury over the medial joint line, overlying skin becomes warm and moist.
2. Fluctuation test and patellar tap test are positive. Hemarthrosis may accompany cruciate tear, meniscus tear, intra-articular fracture.

Special Tests
Special tests may not be possible in the presence of effusion.

Chronic Stage

Chronic Lesion without Effusion
1. Patient with chronic meniscus injury complains of intermittent giving way or locking of the knee followed by effusion. Patient learns to reduce and unlock the joint following which pain gets relieved and movement gets restored. Quadriceps atrophy, more of vastus medialis, is one of the significant findings and weakness is also present.

2. Active and passive joint range of motion is full. Joint play demonstrates pain during external rotation of tibia.
3. McMurray test, Apley test, Helfet test are positive.
4. Joint line tenderness is present over the site of injury.
5. Magnetic resonance imaging (MRI) and arthroscopy confirms the diagnosis.

Management

Factors such as severity of symptoms, ability to perform one's activity, etc. determines whether the injury can be managed conservatively or by surgery. The individual with locked knee, debilitating pain, recurrent mild symptoms of pain, swelling and functional impairment with clinical or MRI evidence of meniscus tear is an indication of surgery. The individual with insignificant symptom, no locking can be managed conservatively.

Conservatively following manipulation to reduce the displaced torn meniscus, pressure bandage to reduce swelling with brace or post-slab immobilization to prevent further damage are given. Keep the part in elevation and apply ice 20 minutes 5 times per day for 48 hours to reduce swelling and resolve acute inflammation.

Cyriax's manipulation, patient in supine lying with the hip and knee flexed to 90° and therapist's one hand is placed at the outer side of the knee joint and other hand at the ankle. Apply strong valgus strain to open the medial side of the joint and gradually extend the knee while rotating it to and fro rapidly. Once reduction is achieved full extension will be restored.

Static quadriceps exercise, high voltage pulsed galvanic stimulation/strong faradic stimulation/Interferential therapy (IFT) is given to reduce swelling, resolve acute inflammation, promote healing, facilitate muscle contraction and relief pain.

Range of motion (ROM) exercise as pain allows, which will promote resolution of effusion, reduce pain, facilitate nourishment to the joint, prevent adhesion formation, maintain joint range of motion, applies optimal stress over the healing tissues for more physiological healing without scar formation.

Straight leg raised, multi-range quadriceps exercise, CKC exercises, once no swelling, no pain and full ROM are achieved, then PRE for muscle strengthening, stretching, endurance exercises are given and full weight-bearing is allowed. Then balance training followed by running program is given once quadriceps and hamstrings strength become 70–80% of the sound side. Patient gradually returns back to activities.

No forced extension in locked knee should be tried. In the presence of locked knee or effusion nonweight-bearing regime must be followed.

LASER can be used meniscal repair. The actual theory underlying the welding phenomenon is not understood completely. Covalent cross-linking or non-covalent electrostatic interactions may occur after heat-induced alterations take place in 3-dimensional structure of collagen molecules.

The surgical intervention of choice in meniscus injury has been excision. This however can result in alteration in knee joint function, reduction in joint space, osteophyte formation, alteration in shape of femoral condyle, i.e. early degeneration of the joint. Therefore, surgical repair of the injured meniscus is the growing trend in orthopedics. Tears in the vascular zone of the meniscus are suitable for repair. Partial meniscectomy is indicated in irreparably damaged meniscus.

Meniscus Repair

The first documented repair of a torn meniscus occurred in 1883 by Thomas Annadale. Meniscal repair become the accepted treatment for certain types of injuries nearly 100 years since Annadale's initial report. In 1989, DeHaven reported on patients treated with open meniscal repair with a rate of healing greater than 85% clinically. Tears in the peripheral third of the meniscus, up to 3 mm can be managed by repair. Intact circumferential hoop fibers heal better than complete radial tear. Radial tear at the posterior horn heals better than those in the middle part. Chronic bucket handle tear that are complex with radial components have more difficulty in healing with repair than simple acute bucket handle tear. Meniscus repair has been found to be more successful when done in conjunction with an ACL reconstruction. Physiotherapy following meniscus repair is important for the successful rehabilitation of the patient so that he can return back to activities after about 6 months.

Early Mobilization Protocol

Phase I: Maximum Protection Phase (for 3 weeks)

Maximum protection to the reparative site is provided while allowing early motion—active assisted/passive movement in 30–80° range with the hinged brace. Terminal 30° knee extension is very complex, external rotation during this range may put undue stress at the reparative site, so should be avoided for 3 weeks.

Nonweight-bearing crutch gait can be allowed. Maximum muscle contraction in the initial phase should be limited due to the dynamic 'F' placed on the meniscus. Aggressive strengthening and ROM exercises, weight-bearing may lead to chronic synovitis, which leads to pain, muscle inhibition, weakness and also delayed healing.

Active submaximal hip exercises, SLR in all directions with the knee brace and submaximal isometric quadriceps exercise, 10 repetitions every hourly.

ROM exercise by continuous passive motion (CPM) with the hinged brace 5–10 minutes every hourly to maintain articular structure nourishment, reduce effusion, pain, apply optimal stress at the reparative site, prevent capsular contracture, etc.

Patellar mobilization and electrical stimulation to quadriceps, particularly vastus medialis oblique (VMO) can be given.

Phase-II: Moderate Protection Phase (after 3–4 weeks)

Range of motion (ROM) and strengthening exercises and weight-bearing is allowed in this phase.

Slowly controlled and increasing flexion-extension by 10°/week. So that 0–120° range is achieved by 8th week. Occasionally, intense exercise will be required to regain extension past 10°.

For strengthening, progressive resisted SLR to hip flexors, extensors, abductors and adductors are given. If resisted SLR is tolerated, isotonic knee exercise can be started. Isotonic, 30–90° knee extension followed by hamstrings exercise can be started after 6 weeks.

For endurance, cycling, swimming, step up, etc. should be given cautiously so that no pain or effusion develop.

Weight-bearing can be initiated after 4 weeks and full weight-bearing by 8th week provided no swelling, no pain, full ROM with adequate strength is achieved.

Balance training: Trauma, surgery and immobilization can alter the mechano-reception in the area of involvement, as a result patient complaint of giving way. Balance training can be given once full weight-bearing is allowed. Wobble board is used for balance training. To start with training is given inside the parallel bars with the eyes open and hand support, with the eyes open and without hand support, with the eyes closed and hand support, with the eyes closed and without hand support, same is repeated outside the parallel bars.

Phase III: Light Activity (8th–12th to 24th weeks, total 12 weeks)

No running, rotational activity or jumping is allowed. Warn against the potential risk of reinjury in returning to early activity.

To improve flexibility, stretching of hamstrings, quadriceps, hip adductors, ITB, TA, etc., for strengthening, isotonic and isokinetic PRE exercises and for endurance, progressive walking to start with 8-10 mm walk add 2 min/week till 20–25 minutes.

Phase IV: Return to Activity (after 24 weeks)

Criterion to start phase IV, there should be no pain in activity, no swelling, full joint ROM, quadriceps and hamstrings strength 70-80% of sound side and no difficulty in stair climbing.

Running, running with turning, running in figure of '8' path, circle running, running with sharp cut and gradually return to sports.

Immobilization Protocol

Two weeks of plaster immobilization with the knee in extension is followed by limited motion (10-80) for another 2 weeks. After that unrestricted motion is allowed.

Arthroscopic Surgery

Postoperative Physiotherapy

Phase I (3–5 days):
1. Rest with compression bandage and elevation, ice therapy 20 minutes 5/6 times per day.
   - Static quadriceps (Fig. 3.4) and high voltage pulsed galvanic stimulation (Fig. 3.5)/strong faradic stimulation/interferential therapy.

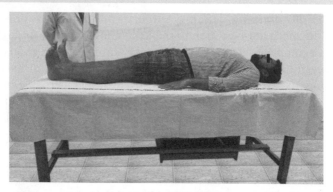

Fig. 3.4: Static quadriceps.

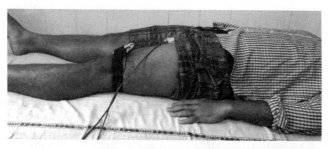

Fig. 3.5: Strong faradic stimulation to vastus medialis oblique (VMO).

  – Active ankle foot toe movements
  – Active hip movements in all directions with the brace.
2. Once SLR possible, active knee movement started after 2–3 days.

Phase II (5–15 days):
1. ROM exercise 0–90°
2. Progressive resisted SLR
3. CKC exercises such as leg press (Fig. 3.6) or by the use of resistance band (Fig. 3.7), step-up, etc.
4. Endurance training such as swimming, cycling (Fig. 3.8), rowing, etc.
5. Partial weight-bearing crutch walking can be initiated.

Phase–III (15–21 days):
1. Vigorous PRE for the hip
2. For ROM-squat, prone kneel to sitting, etc.
3. Stretching of hamstrings (Fig. 3.9), quadriceps, hip adductors (Fig. 3.10), ITB, TA (Fig. 3.11), etc.

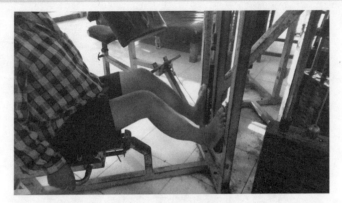

Fig. 3.6: Leg press.

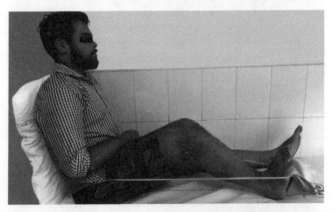

Fig. 3.7: Close kinetic chain knee extension exercise using resistance band.

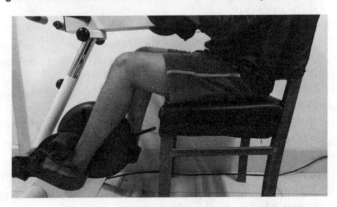

Fig. 3.8: Static cycling.

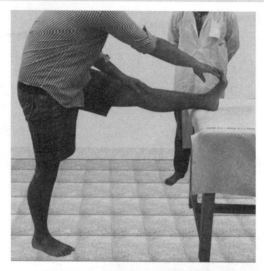

Fig. 3.9: Hamstring stretching in standing.

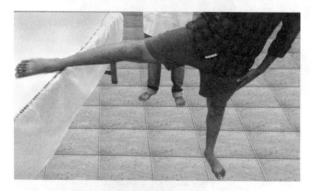

Fig. 3.10: Streching of hip adductors.

4. Endurance training and CKC exercises continued
5. Full weight-bearing is allowed.

Phase IV (4–6 weeks):

1. Progressive strengthening (Fig. 3.12), stretching, endurance training continued.
2. Balance training can be initiated
3. Running program given once quadriceps and hamstrings strength 70–80% of sound side.
4. Return to activities after 6 weeks.

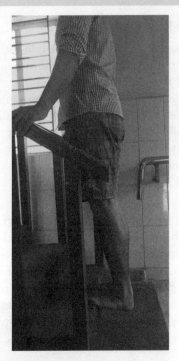

Fig. 3.11: Stretching of gastrocnemius.

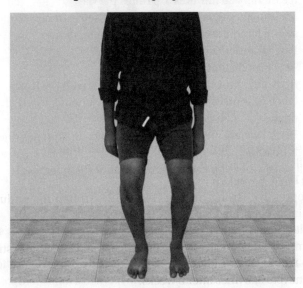

Fig. 3.12: Mini squat.

Complications of Meniscal Repair

Other than the failure of a repaired meniscus to heal, the complication rate after meniscal repair is low. Stiffness is a complication occasionally seen after meniscal repair, with a prevalence ranging from 6–12%. Stiffness can be decreased by positioning the knee near full extension when medial meniscus is repaired and by using an accelerated rehabilitation program when medial meniscus repair is performed in conjunction with ACL reconstruction. There may be neurovascular injury also.

Meniscectomy

Oblique incision starts close to inferomedial aspect of patella, extends downwards and backwards to a point 1 cm below the joint line. Skin, subcutaneous tissues, capsule, synovial membrane are cut, it may involve infrapatellar branch of saphenous nerve.

Transverse incision of 4 cm length over anteromedial aspect of knee parallel to articular surface of tibia about 1 cm above it. Disadvantage of this incision is scar adherent to the surface of tibia.

1. Postoperatively, rest with compression bandage and elevation for 2/3 days.
   - Ice therapy 20 minutes 5/6 times per day.
   - Static quadriceps and high voltage pulsed galvanic stimulation/ strong faradic stimulation/Interferential therapy
   - Patellar mobilization.
   - Active ankle foot toe movements.
   - Active hip movements in all directions with the brace.
   - Once SLR possible, active knee movement started after 2–3 days.
   - Partial weight-bearing with knee brace in crutches once SLR is possible.
2. Full weight-bearing can be initiated after stitch removal.

Replacement of Meniscus

Indicated in cases where meniscus tears cannot be successfully repaired. Meniscus transplantation has been shown to be an acceptable procedure for younger patients. The primary candidate is a patient younger than age 50 years who has had a total meniscectomy and who either has pain in the tibiofemoral component, arthroscopic evidence of articular cartilage deterioration or both.[10,11]

Mesenchymal Stem Cells in Meniscus Repair

Tissue engineering of meniscus with mesenchymal-based cells seems to be a promising approach to treat meniscal tears and defects in order to restore as much native meniscal tissue as possible.[9]

CRUCIATE LIGAMENT INJURY

Anterior cruciate ligament originates from anterior intercondylar area of tibia runs backward, upward and laterally to the medial aspect of lateral femoral condyle in the intercondylar notch. It checks forward displacement of tibia over femur, extension of the knee and internal rotation of tibia on femur.

Posterior cruciate ligament originates from posterior intercondylar area of tibia runs forward, upward and medially to the lateral aspect of medial femoral condyle in the intercondylar notch. It checks backward displacement of tibia, extension of the knee and internal rotation of tibia on femur. During squatting forward gliding of femur on tibia is checked by PCL and popliteus.

Anterolaterally, lateral patellar retinaculum and ITB checks excessive internal rotation of tibia and posterolaterally biceps femoris tendon checks excessive internal rotation and anterior displacement of tibia. They reinforce the cruciates.

Anterior to posterior displacement of tibia as occurs due to falling on the knees, i.e. proximal end of tibia or due to dash-board injury results in injury PCL. A force against the anterior thigh, which can drive femur backward on the tibia, while the knee is close to full extension, tends to stress the ACL. Forced internal rotation may result in isolated injury of ACL. Hyperextension injury results in tearing of posterior capsule followed by ACL and then PCL (Fig. 3.13). Noncontact mechanisms were classified as sudden deceleration prior to a change of direction or landing motion, while contact injuries occurred as a result of valgus collapse of the knee.[12]

Several intrinsic and extrinsic risk factors of ACL injury have been found. The two most established intrinsic risk factors are increased tibial plateau slope and a narrow intercondylar notch. Many other potential intrinsic factors have been noted such as joint laxity, familial predisposition, and body mass index (BMI), to name a few. Shoe-surface interface and position of play have been found to be extrinsic risk factors of ACL injury.

Injury to ACL is potentially crippling, affecting active people both young and old. The incidence is more common in competitive sports such as football, skiing, and soccer. It is reported that 70% of acute ACL injuries are sports related, involving recreational and high-performance athletes. Female athletes with increased dynamic valgus and high abduction loads are at increased risk of ACL injury.[13] Chronic ACL deficiency results in significant knee instability, secondary damage to other knee structures and early degenerative arthritis.

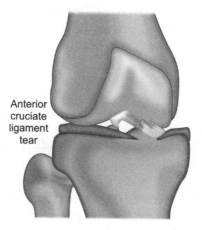

Anterior cruciate ligament tear

Fig. 3.13: Anterior cruciate ligament tear.
(*Source:* eOrthopod. 2006. http://www.orthogate.org/).

Patient develops joint effusion and pain following injury. As the initial swelling and pain subsides, patient complaint of instability of the knee. The knee buckles into hyperextension in chronic posterolateral instability. Functionally, patient finds difficulty in descending stairs, squatting, running with sudden stop, etc. activities. Patient walks with the knee in flexion to avoid instability. There may be varus thrust while walking, which may lead to instability with cutting activities.

Anterior-posterior translation is checked at 30° and 90° of knee flexion. Slight increase posterior translation at 30° but not at 90° indicates posterolateral injury, increased posterior translation at both 30° and 90° indicates injury to PCL (Fig. 3.14). Active posterior drawer

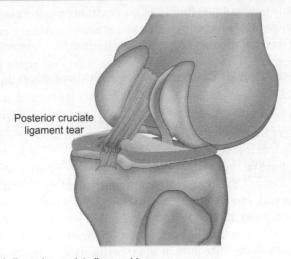

Posterior cruciate
ligament tear

Fig. 3.14: Posterior cruciate ligament tear.

Source: Kiritsis PA. Patient's guide to posterior cruciate ligament injuries. http://www. kneeandshouldersurgery.com

test, Lachman test, etc. demonstrate increased anterior-posterior translation and external rotation recurvatum test, posterolateral drawer test, etc. demonstrate posterolateral instability.

Intercondylar notch stenosis has also been considered an intrinsic risk factor of ACL injury. Other potential intrinsic risk factors of ACL injury identified by 2 systematic reviews include: ACL geometry in females, foot pronation, pelvic tilt, generalized joint laxity, anterior knee laxity in females, menstrual cycle phase, dynamic knee valgus and knee flexor/extensor preactivation in females, familial predisposition, and the presence of collagen type I alpha 1 *(COL1A1)* gene, height, and BMI.[14,15]

Prevention of Cruciate Injuries

1. Dry weather conditions, artificial turf, and increased posterior tibial slope were associated with increased risk of ACL injury in males.[16-18]
2. The general principles of rehabilitation of ligamentous injuries are as follows:
    - The deleterious effects of immobilization must be minimized.
    - Healing tissue must not be overstressed.

- The patient must fulfill certain criteria to progress from one stage of rehabilitation to the next stage.
- The rehabilitation program must be based on biomechanics.

Biomechanics of Exercise in the Rehabilitation of ACL and PCL

The ACL is often considered the most important stabilizer of the joint. Its primary role is to prevent anterior tibial translation at the knee, particularly at low flexion angles.[19]

The hamstrings (biceps femoris, semitendinosus, semi-membranosus) are technically antagonists of the quadriceps, opposing knee extensor moments. In closed-chain exercise, however, they behave paradoxically and co-contract with the quadriceps. This synergistic action has important implications for enhancing the integrity of the knee joint in squat performance. Specifically, the hamstrings exert a counter regulatory pull on the tibia, helping to neutralize the anterior tibiofemoral shear imparted by the quadriceps and thus alleviating stress on the ACL.[19,20]

Kaufman et al. reported that, posterior shear force during open kinetic chain resisted knee extension changes to anterior shear at 50–55° of extension. Kaufman et al. reported a linear relationship between posterior shear force and knee flexion angle during open kinetic chain resisted knee flexion. From 0–50° of knee flexion posterior shear force was reported below 1 × BW whereas from 50–90° of knee flexion the force increased to 1.7 × BW then sharply declined again at 100° of knee flexion.

Brown et al. reviewed 6 studies and determined that there were differences between planned and unplanned side stepping tasks, especially for loading associated with weight acceptance rather than during push-off. The authors recommended that unplanned tasks should be incorporated into screening and injury prevention training programs.

During closed kinetic chain exercise posterior shear force increases linearly with knee flexion, but the magnitude is less than that during open kinetic chain (OKC) knee flexion. The hamstrings have the potential of negating the anterior tibial translation caused by quadriceps during closed-chain kinetic exercises.

Lutz reported posterior shear force 939N at 30° of knee flexion during maximal isometric knee flexion contraction when compared to a maximum anterior shear force 285N at 30° of knee flexion during maximal isometric knee extension contraction.

Markolf and coworkers reported that passive extension of knee generates forces in the ACL only during last 10° of extension; at 5° of hyperextension mean force was 118N.

To minimize posterior shear over the PCL, OKC knee extension should be performed initially from 60° to 0°, CKC front squat or leg press should be performed from 0° to 60° and OKC knee flexion should be avoided.

Partial cruciate tear, negative Lachman test, older persons with complete tear and low activity level can be managed conservatively. Complete tear, physiologically young persons with high level of activity or with associated collateral rupture and/or repairable meniscal tear require surgery. Primary cruciate ligament repair with/without augmentation, intra-articular reconstruction by using autograft, allograft or prosthetic ligament with/without extra-articular stabilization are various surgical procedures for the management of cruciate deficient knee. Patellar tendon, semitendinosus, gracilis and ITB are used as autograft for the reconstruction. A variety of graft fixation methods exist including staples, suture over buttons, interference screws and screws with spiked soft tissue washers. Screw with spiked washer or spiked soft tissue plate is the commonly used fixation method. Intra-articular reconstruction by using central one-third of patellar tendon autograft is the method of choice in ACL reconstruction.

Nonoperative Posterior Cruciate Ligament Rehabilitation

Maximum Protection Phase (for 3 weeks)

1. Rest with compression, elevation, protection by knee brace and ice 20 minutes 5–6 times/day for 48 hours.
2. Range of motion exercise 0-60° by the CPM will help to reduce effusion and pain, articular structure nourishment, apply optimal stress at the reparative site, prevent capsular contracture, etc.
3. Active ankle foot and toes movements and SLR for hip flexion, abduction and adduction.
4. Static quadriceps exercises, patellar mobilization and electrical stimulation to quadriceps, particularly VMO can be given.
5. Open kinetic chain (OKC) knee extension should be performed initially from 60° to 0°, CKC front squat or leg press should be

performed from 0° to 45° and multiangle isometric quadriceps exercise at 60°, 40°, and 20°.
6. Weight-bearing with crutches can be initiated after a few days.

Moderate Protection Phase (3–6 weeks)

1. Knee brace is replaced by functional brace
2. Progressive ROM and stretching exercises as tolerated by the patient.
3. Progressive resisted knee extension from 60° to 0°, aggressive CKC squat or leg press from 0° to 60° and multiangle isometric quadriceps exercise at 60°, 40°, and 20° are performed to improve lower extremity strength.

Minimum Protection Phase (6–12 weeks)

1. Strengthening, stretching and endurance exercises are performed, balance training can be started.
2. Running program can be initiated once there is no swelling, no pain, no laxity and isokinetic evaluation shows quadriceps and hamstrings strength 70–80% of the sound side. Then gradually patient returns back to activities.

Rehabilitation Following PCL Reconstruction

Knee bracing: There is no evidence that braces contribute to pain control, graft stability, ROM, or protection from additional injury.[21-23]

Immediate Postoperative Phase (1 week)

1. Rest with compression, elevation, protection by knee brace locked at 0° of extension and ice 20 minutes 5–6 times/day for 48 hours.
2. Range of motion exercise 0–60° by the CPM will help to reduce effusion and pain, articular structure nourishment, apply optimal stress at the reparative site, prevent capsular contracture, etc.
3. Active ankle foot and toes movements and SLR for hip flexion, abduction and adduction.
4. Static quadriceps exercises, patellar mobilization and electrical stimulation to quadriceps, particularly VMO can be given.
5. Weight-bearing with the brace locked and with a pair of crutches as tolerated by the patient.

Maximum Protection Phase (2–3 weeks)

1. Intermittent ROM exercise 0° to 60°
2. OKC knee extension should be performed initially from 60° to 0°, CKC front squat or leg press should be performed from 0–45° and multiangle isometric quadriceps exercise at 60°, 40°, and 20°.
3. Static quadriceps exercises, patellar mobilization and electrical stimulation to quadriceps, particularly VMO can be given.
4. Weight-bearing with crutches as tolerated.

Moderate Protection Phase (3–6 weeks)

1. Knee brace is locked at 0° of extension and weight-bearing without crutches can be started.
2. Progressive ROM 0–90° and stretching exercises as tolerated by the patient.
3. Progressive resisted knee extension from 60° to 0°, CKC squat or leg press from 0° to 45° and multiangle isometric quadriceps exercise at 60°, 40°, and 20° are performed to improve lower extremity strength.
4. Initiate cycling to improve endurance.

Minimum Protection Phase/Controlled Ambulation Phase (6–12 weeks)

1. Knee brace is replaced by functional brace and walking with the brace open allowed.
2. Progressive strengthening, stretching and endurance exercises are performed.
3. Initiate swimming and balance training.

Light Activity Phase (3–6 months)

1. Progressive strengthening, stretching, endurance exercises and balance training are continued.
2. Running program can be initiated once there is no swelling, no pain, no laxity and isokinetic evaluation shows quadriceps and hamstrings strength 70–80% of the sound side. Then plyometrics can be initiated and gradually patient returns back to activities after 6 months.

Nonoperative Anterior Cruciate Ligament Rehabilitation

Nonoperative management of ACL injury may be indicated for those who have an isolated injury without damage to other structures and willing to modify the lifestyles that cause instability. The aim of treatment following ACL injury is early resolution of inflammation, restoration of ROM, regaining muscle strength and prevention from further damage.

Cold compression is given to reduce swelling and pain. ROM exercises are performed to restore motion. ROM improves with as swelling and pain subsides. Failure to regain movement particularly extension, may indicate a torn meniscus and require further evaluation. Isometric quadriceps and hamstrings exercises should be initiated to prevent muscle atrophy. Ambulation with knee brace and crutches is allowed, which is discontinued once full knee extension without quadriceps lag and walking without any deviation are regained.

More aggressive physiotherapy can begin once swelling and pain subsides, and full ROM is regained. The emphasis should be given on improving the strength and endurance of the muscles that cross the knee, particularly hamstrings and gastrocnemius, which pull the tibia posteriorly. Open kinetic progressive hamstrings strengthening exercise can be used. Standing heel raises can be used to develop gastrocnemius muscle. Closed kinetic exercises can be used to develop strength and endurance of the muscles of lower extremity in functional pattern while minimizing patellofemoral stresses. Closed kinetic exercises are progressed as tolerated and may include wall slides, mini squats, step-ups and leg press. Cycling and swimming helps to improve endurance of lower extremity muscles. Use of toe clips and pedaling with one leg increases hamstrings activity.

Once strength and endurance of lower extremity muscles have been established, it is necessary to develop neuromuscular control to enhance dynamic stability of the knee. Balance training is followed by progressive activity training. Gradually patient progresses from walking to jogging, running, sprinting, acceleration-deceleration, jumping, cutting, pivoting and twisting. Use of a functional knee brace may be helpful as the returns to activity.

Rehabilitation Following Anterior Cruciate Ligament Repair

Primary repair of with/without augmentation is indicated in persons with proximal ACL tear in conjunction with rupture of patellar tendon, complete dislocation of knee with rupture of most of the ligamentous structure around the joint. Primary repair with/without augmentation has a markedly decreased likelihood of success, if used to repair middle, distal or combined tears of the ACL. Accelerated rehabilitation, early weight bearing, and early ROM exercises are likely safe and possibly beneficial to patient outcomes.[23]

Cryotherapy is safe and effective during the short-term postoperative period. Cryotherapy was statistically significantly associated with reduced pain but was not significantly associated with ROM or postoperative drainage output.[24,25]

The knee is taken through full ROM on the operating table to ensure that full motion is available. Following wound closure hinged brace is applied and continuous passive motion is begun in the brace. Passive knee extension and active knee flexion can be allowed on first postoperative day. From 6 to 16 weeks, patient continues to bend the knee in full range with the hamstrings, lay in prone position with the foot out of the bed for gravity-assisted passive knee extension, static cycling and walk inside the hydrotherapy pool. Active knee extension beyond 45° should not be permitted for at least 6 months. In case of persistent instability, the period may be extended from 6 to 12 months. Progressive-resisted exercises by using elastic resistance bands should be done to improve muscle strength (Fig. 3.15).

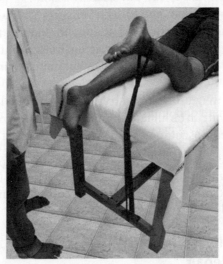

Fig. 3.15: Hamstring strengthening by resistance band.

Rehabilitation Following Anterior Cruciate Ligament Reconstruction

Maximum Protection Phase (for 6 weeks)

1. Rest with compression, elevation, protection by knee brace locked in extension or slight flexion and ice 20 minutes 5–6 times/day for 48 hours.

2. The stress on the graft is maximum from 20° to 0° extension. But in case of isolated intra-articular ACL reconstruction full extension can be done without disrupting the autograft, patellar tendon graft. The hinged brace is locked at 0° of extension. The brace is unlocked and ROM exercise from 0° to 90° by the CPM can be given, which helps to reduce effusion and pain, articular structure nourishment, apply optimal stress at the reparative site to reorient the collagen tissues, proper vascularization of the graft, create stronger healing ligament, prevent capsular contracture, etc. In case of semitendinosus or ITB or synthetic graft exercises and weight-bearing should be done more cautiously.

   – But in case of combined extra-articular procedure, collateral ligament reconstruction and meniscus repair, the knee must be immobilized in 20–30° of knee flexion.

   – Active ankle foot and toes movements, SLR for hip flexion, extension, abduction and adduction, static quadriceps and hamstrings exercises, electrical stimulation can be given to prevent disuse atrophy. Patellar mobilization should be given.

   – Partial weight-bearing with crutches and brace locked at 0° of extension can be initiated from the 1st/2nd postoperative day. But in case of combined procedure, it is deferred by 7–10 days.

   – CKC squat or leg press 0–60° and multiangle isometric quadriceps and hamstrings exercise at 60°, 40°, and 20° can be started after 7–10 days.

   – By 4 weeks the bone graft are healed and vascularization is beginning. By 9 weeks vascularization is well established. Therefore after 9 weeks exercises can be more vigorous.

– Full weight-bearing with brace locked at 0° of extension can be initiated after 3 weeks, but in case of combined procedure full weight-bearing is allowed after 6 weeks.

Moderate Protection Phase (6–12 weeks)

1. Full weight-bearing with brace locked at 0° of extension is possible. After 9 weeks functional knee brace can be used during weight-bearing activities.
2. Progressive stretching, ROM, strengthening and endurance exercises are performed. Balance training can be started.

Minimum Protection Phase/Controlled Ambulation Phase (12–20 weeks)

1. Knee brace is removed.
2. Progressive strengthening, stretching endurance exercises and balance training are continued. Proprioceptive and balance training were associated with improvements in knee joint position sense, muscle strength, perceived knee function, and hop testing in ACL-deficient knees. ACL-deficient knees showed significant improvements in knee function, function for activities of daily living, and single-leg hop testing and decreased instability after neuromuscular and proprioceptive training.[26, 27]
3. Running program can be initiated once there is no swelling, no pain, no laxity and isokinetic evaluation shows quadriceps and hamstrings strength 70–80% of the sound side.
4. Plyomerics can be initiated after 20 weeks. Then gradually patient returns back to activities after 6 months.

Complications of surgery include adhesions, decreased motion, decreased strength of quadriceps and hamstrings, graft failure, loss of proprioception, etc.

REFERENCES

1. Chen L, et al. medial collateral ligament injuries of the knee: current treatment concepts. Curr Rev musculoskelet Med. 2008;1(2):108-13.
2. Indelicato PA. Isolated medial collateral ligament injuries in the knee. Jam Acad Orthop Surg. 1995. 3(1):9-14.

3. Gardener JC, Weiss JA, Rosenberg TD. Strain in human collateral ligament during valgus loading of the knee. Clin Orthop Relat Res. 2001;391: 266-74.

4. Giannotti BF, Rudy T, Graziano J. The non-surgical management of isolated medial collateral ligament injuries of the knee. Sports Med Arthrosc. 2006;14(2):74-7.

5. DeGrace DM. Analysis of medial collateral ligament injuries of the knee. The Harvard Orthopaedic Journal. 2013;15.

6. Cimino PM. The incidence of meniscal tears associated with acute anterior cruciate ligament disruption secondary to snow skiing accidents. Arthroscopy. 1994;10:198-200.

7. Binfield PM, Maffulli N, King JB. Patterns of meniscal tears associated with anterior cruciate ligament lesions in athletes. Injury. 1993;24: 557-61.

8. Nag H, et al. Meniscus injury and management: All India Institute of Medical Sciences, New Delhi, India. JIMSA. 2011;24 No. 1.

9. Angele P, et al. Role of mesenchymal stem cells in meniscal repair. Journal of Experimental Orthopaedics. 2014;1:12.

10. Hannink G, Buma P, et al. Meniscus replacement using synthetic materials. Clin Sports Med. 2009;28:143-56.

11. Pasa L, Pokorny V, Kalandra S, Melichar I, Bilik A. Transplantation of deep frozen menisci. Acta Chir Orthop Traumatol Cech. 2008;75:40-7.

12. Boden PB, Dean GS, Feagin JA, et al. Mechanisms of anterior cruciate ligament injury. Healio Orthopedics. 2000; 23 (6):573-8.

13. Timothy E, et al. Biomechanical measures of neuromuscular control and valgus loading of the knee predict anterior cruciate ligament injury risk in female athletes—a prospective study. Am J Sports Med. 2005;33(4): 492-501.

14. Serpell BG, Scarvell JM, Ball NB, Smith PN. Mechanisms and risk factors for noncontact ACL injury in age mature athletes who engage in field or court sports: a summary of the literature since 1980. J Strength Cond Res. 2012;26:3160-76.

15. Posthumus M, Collins M, September AV, Schwellnus MP. The intrinsic risk factors for ACL ruptures: an evidence-based review. Phys Sports-med. 2011;39:62-73.

16. Klein K. The deep squat exercise as utilized in weight training for athletes and its effects on the ligaments of the knee. J Assoc Phys Ment Rehabil. 1961;15:6-11.

17. Alentorn-Geli E, Mendiguchi´a J, Samuelsson K, et al. Prevention of anterior cruciate ligament injuries in sports. Part I: systematic review of risk factors in male athletes. Knee Surg Sports Traumatol Arthrosc. 2014;22:3-15.

18. Sadoghi P, von Keudell A, Vavken P. Effectiveness of anterior cruciate ligament injury prevention training programs. J Bone Joint Surg Am. 2012;94:769-76.

19. Escamilla RF. Knee biomechanics of the dynamic squat exercise. Med Sci Sports Exerc. 2001;33:127-41.
20. Rasch PJ, Burke RK. Kinesiology and Applied Anatomy, (5th edition). Philadelphia, PA: Lea and Febiger; 1974.
21. Kruse LM, Gray B, Wright RW. Rehabilitation after anterior cruciate ligament reconstruction: a systematic review. J Bone Joint Surg Am. 2012;94:1737-48.
22. Wright RW, Fetzer GB. Bracing after ACL reconstruction: a systematic review. Clin Orthop Relat Res. 2007;455:162-8.
23. Wright RW, Preston E, Fleming BC, et al. A systematic review of anterior cruciate ligament reconstruction rehabilitation: Part I. Continuous passive motion, early weight bearing, postoperative bracing, and home-based rehabilitation. J Knee Surg. 2008;21:217-24.
24. Martimbianco AL, Gomes da Silva BN, de Carvalho AP, et al. Effectiveness and safety of cryotherapy after arthroscopic anterior cruciate ligament reconstruction. A systematic review of the literature. Phys Ther Sport. 2014;15:261-8.
25. Raynor MC, Pietrobon R, Guller U, et al. Cryotherapy after ACL reconstruction: a meta-analysis. J Knee Surg. 2005;18:123-9.
26. Cooper RL, Taylor NF, Feller JA. A systematic review of the effect of proprioceptive and balance exercises on people with an injured or reconstructed anterior cruciate ligament. Res Sports Med. 2005;13:163-78.
27. Zech A, Hubscher M, Vogt L, et al. Neuromuscular training for rehabilitation of sports injuries: a systematic review. Med Sci Sports Exerc. 2009;41:1831-41.

Chapter 4

Common Arthritic Conditions

OSTEOARTHRITIS OF KNEE

Osteoarthritis (Fig. 4.1) is the most common joint disorder causing disability affecting more than millions of people all over the world. More disability and clinical symptoms result from osteoarthritis of knee joint than from any other joint. Osteoarthritis of the knee joint is reported to be a major health problem faced by most of the population currently. Its prevalence after the age of 65 years is about 60% in male and 70% in female. Osteoarthritis/degenerative joint disease of the knee may occur in the medial and/or lateral compartment of tibiofemoral joint and/or patellofemoral joint (TFJ/PFJ). The PFJ is one of the most commonly affected compartments. The PFJ is involved either in isolation or in combination with the TFJ in 49% of all cases of knee osteoarthritis. Isolated patellofemoral osteoarthritis is relatively rare. Investigation in people with knee pain revealed

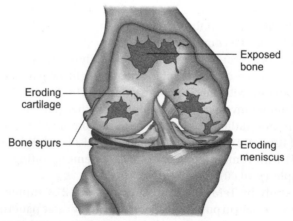

Fig. 4.1: Osteoarthritis.
(*Source:* Oxford University Hospitals. http://www.ouh.nhs.uk).

the most common radiographic pattern to be a combined TFJ and PFJ disease. Individuals with combined PFJ and TFJ OA had more symptoms, lower function in sports and recreation and worse knee related quality than individuals with isolated TFJ OA.

World Health Organization (WHO) estimates that 10% of the world's population over the age of 60 years suffers from OA and that 80% of people with OA have limitation of movement and 25% cannot perform the major daily activities. OA is major cause of impairment and disability in elderly and poses a significant economic burden in the community.

Epidemiology, Prevalence and Incidence

Osteoarthritis is a globally common joint disorder with symptoms of pain, joint stiffness and reduced function. Amongst the elderly it accounts for more disability than any other disease. Nearly one in five women over the age of 60 years is affected (46) and 60% of people over the age of 64 years have moderate to severe OA in at least one joint. The prevalence of OA rises with age, and with increasing longevity, the incidence is certain to rise. A paper published in 1995 in the US suggested that by the year 2020, there will be a 66% increase in the number of people with OA related disability.

Traditionally knee OA has been viewed primarily as a disorder of the TFJ as radiographic assessment has tended to focus only on the anteroposterior X-ray which does not image the PFJ. As the use of lateral and skyline X-rays has increased, so to have awareness of the PFJ involvement in the OA process. In fact the PFJ is the most commonly affected compartment.

Authors of a recent community-based study of knee OA observed a higher frequency of radiographic osteophytes in the patellofemoral joint compared with the TFJ compartment (218/334 vs.184/334, p <0.01). Another investigation in people with knee pain revealed the most common radiographic pattern to be combined TFJ and PFJ disease (40%, 314/777 subjects) followed by isolated PFJ OA (24%, 186/777) with remaining 32% (246/777) demonstrating normal radiographs (p <0.001).

In a study by TeMcAindon, Snow et al. in 273 subjects who reported knee pain in postal questionnaire survey three patterns were predominant patellofemoral, medial, and medial/patellofemoral joint disease in 11, 21, and 7% of the men and in 24, 12, and 6% of women. The occurrence of isolated symptomatic patellofemoral joint OA in this sample aged more than 55 years was estimated as 8% in women and 2% in men.

The prevalence of radiographic knee OA rises in women from 1% to 4% in those aged 24–45 years to 53% in those 80 years and older. In men, the prevalence rises from 1% to 6% in those 45 years and younger to 22% to 33% in those 80 years and older.

PATELLOFEMORAL DYSFUNCTION

There are two common dysfunctions of the patellofemoral joint-patella becoming too compressed against the femur and moving too far laterally in the intercondylar groove. Both conditions cause abrasion of the cartilage, leading to inflammation and degeneration. It becomes too compressed due to increased flexion of the knee, which is caused by sustained tension in the hamstrings, iliotibial band (ITB), and gastrocnemius or by a shortened joint capsule. This compression force is dramatically increased when a person climbs stairs or gets up from chair.

If the patella is compressed laterally in the trochlear groove, it is called patellar tracking dysfunction. The resultant of quadriceps muscle force in the frontal plane faces upward and outward. Therefore with active quadriceps contraction patella tracks upward and outward. With increase in Q-angle, there is more risk of lateral tracking and subluxation. Lateral subluxation of patella is prevented by anterior prominence of femoral condyle, deep patellar groove and dynamically by the force of contraction of vastus medialis obliquus. Genu valgus, ITB tightness, femoral anteversion, external tibial torsion, foot pronation, high riding small patella, weakness of vastus medialis, an over development of the vastus lateralis, lateral retinaculum, and tensor fascia lata (TFL), etc. are the factors that precipitate to lateral tracking. This restricts the medial glide of patella and increasing the pressure of the patellofemoral joint.

Soft tissue tensions, medial and lateral retinacular, particularly the two distal expansions of the ITB, joint capsule and ligaments all contribute to maintain patella alignment. It has been proposed that a tight ITB through its attachment of the lateral retinaculum into the patella could cause lateral patellar tracking, patella tilt and compression.

It has been well established that shortening of the lateral retinaculum is a common condition in patients with patellofemoral dysfunction. This causes progressive tilting of the patella if the medial static stabilizers are stretched or the dynamic stabilizer (VMO) is weak. This leads to abnormal patellar alignment, i.e. lateral displacement and lateral tilt. As the patellofemoral joint is subjected to elevated stress this causes patellofemoral pain. Medial glide of patella can be used extensively to stretch tight lateral retinaculum.

As the patella tracks laterally, the odd medial facet of patella, which is normally non-articulatory, becomes articulatory. The non-articulatory odd medial facet of patella is soft as it is not subjected to stress. With lateral tracking of patella, the odd medial facet of patella will be subjected to compressive loading and gets traumatized. Each time the knee extends, patella tracks laterally and the lateral PFJ gets compressed and degenerate overtime. Gradually, the lateral patellar retinaculum becomes tight and medial patellar retinaculum will be subjected to tensile stress, so there develops chronic inflammation.

Risk Factor for Patellofemoral Osteoarthritis

Risk factors can be divided into two pathogenic mechanisms. They are systemic factors influencing a generalized predisposition to osteoarthritis and local factors resulting in abnormal biomechanical loading at specific joints.

Systemic factors include person's age, sex, inherited susceptibility to osteoarthritis, and other factors some of which yet to be identified.

Local factors include varus-valgus malalignment, patellar malalignment, anatomical abnormalities, chondromalacia patella, and repetitive use of the joint, including that caused by occupational activities.

The etiopathogenesis of osteoarthritis is widely believed to be the result of local mechanical factors along with the context of systemic susceptibility.

Systemic Factors

Age: The prevalence and incidence of osteoarthritis correlates with age. The increase in osteoarthritis with age is likely a consequence of biological changes which occur with ageing which make it susceptible to disease. These changes include an increased response time in anticipatory and incoming transarticular load and the decrease in muscle strength. In addition chondrocytes, the cells in the cartilage, lose their responsiveness to stimuli for growth factors and cytokines with age, so that a dynamic load that would otherwise lead to a reparative matrix synthesis in cartilage does not do so in older joints. Also, with age, ligaments loosen and cartilage thins, thinning of cartilage increases shear stress at the basal levels where noncalcified cartilage attaches at the tidemark to the calcified layer of cartilage, clefts occur at these attachments, suggesting that excessive stress damages the attachment between cartilage and its base.

The percent of people with evidence of osteoarthritis in one or more joints increases from less than 5% of people between 15 and 44 years, to 25–30% of people 45–64 years of age and to more than 60% and as high as 90% in some population of the people over 65 years of age. Shouten et al. in a 12-year follow-up study of knee osteoarthritis, reported that patients over 60 years of age at baseline had an almost four-fold higher rate of joint space loss than those aged 45–49 years.

More than a third of people over 45 years report joint symptoms that vary from a occasional joint stiffness and intermittent aching associated with activity, to permanent loss of motion and constant deep pain. After age of 40 the incidence of osteoarthritis increases rapidly with each passing decade in all joints and in most joints the incidence is greater in women than in men. Investigation has shown that OA occurs in 44–70% of individuals more than 55 years of age and 10% of them are functionally limited.

Gender: In population based studies, the incidence of patellofemoral OA was common in women 24% versus 12% males. In the Framingham study, 2% of women per year developed radiographic knee OA. In another population-based study in Holland (age of subjects 46-66 years), about 2% of women and 0.8% of men developed radiographic knee OA per year.

Genetic Factors

Osteoarthritis of the knee is considerably less heritable with estimates ranging from no heritability at all to 30% heritability. Heritability for

OA appears to be higher among women than among men for almost all joints.

Obesity: Obesity is associated with an increased risk of knee osteoarthritis specifically at the patellofemoral compartment, at the tibiofemoral compartment and most notably with simultaneous arthritis at both those sites. Obesity is a strong risk factor for subsequent developments of bilateral knee OA in those who already have unilateral OA. Obesity is associated with both symptomatic and asymptomatic knee OA and this association is more pronounced in women. Although elevated BMI increase the risk of knee OA progression, the effect of body mass index (BMI) is limited to knees in which moderate malalignment exists.

Biomechanical Risk Factors

Influence of Patella Alta on Knee Extensor Mechanics

Individuals with patella alta have a more efficient knee extensor mechanism and would be expected to generate similar joint reaction forces per unit quadriceps force compared to subjects with normal patella position.

Therefore, persons with patella alta may experience less PFJ reaction force to overuse the same knee flexion moment in the range of 0–60° of flexion.

Chondromalacia Patella

Patellofemoral joint mechanics demonstrated a strong correlation with the etiology of PFJ disorders, such as chondromalacia. Chondromalacia of the patella is considered the primary precursor to arthrosis of the knee. The cause of chondromalacia of the patella can be any condition in which the normal rhythm of the quadriceps mechanism is disturbed resulting in abnormal stress distribution in the articulating surface of the PFJ. The imbalance of the patellofemoral mediolateral force, often in conjunction with abnormalities in the bony anatomy of the joint, has also been associated with subluxation of the patella, leading to chondromalacia and arthrosis. This type of disorder may result from abnormally high stress on the articular surface of the PFJ caused by angular and torsional deformities of the femur.

Vastus Medialis Obliquus Weakness

The vastus medialis has an important role as a medial stabilizer of the patella and aids in normal functioning of the patellofemoral joint. In cadaver studies Ahmed et al. in 1983 showed that the removal of vastus medialis obliquus (VMO) tendon shifted the pressure zone from the center to the lateral facet of the patella. Similarly Goh et al. in 1995 reported that the absence of VMO caused the load on the lateral patellar facet throughout the range of knee motion.

Varus-Valgus Alignment and Patellar Kinematics in Individuals with Knee OA

Cahue et al. found that valgus alignment is associated with the progression of lateral patellofemoral OA and varus malalignment is associated with the progression of medial patellofemoral OA. Varus or valgus alignment does not always predict the dimension of patellar kinematics. Valgus alignment is associated with hypoplasia of the lateral condyle whereas varus alignment is not associated with hypoplasia of the medial condyle. Varus-valgus laxity at the tibiofemoral joint tends to increase in latter stages of OA as a result of cartilage loss 25 while laxity in other directions may decrease. Hunter et al. 2007 found that baseline knee alignment is not associated with either incident radiographical TF OA or medial TF OA. Malalignment is not a risk factor for OA, but rather is a marker of disease severity and/or its progression.

Q-Angle

Huberti and Hayes documented the effect of an increased Q-angle by measuring patellofemoral contact pressure. It was noted that when the Q-angle was decreased 10° from the normal physiological position increase in contact pressure were observed. Install et al. in a prospective study found that chondromalacia patella were more common in patients with larger Q angles. Messier et al. reported that Q angles were larger in groups with patellofemoral pain.

Patellar Malalignment

According to Gresalmer et al. patella malalignment is a translational or rotational deviation of the patella related to any axis, and it can be a major component of patellar pain in adults. Uncontrolled data suggests that patella are located centrally in the trochlear groove, and not malaligned may be less likely to develop OA. Patellar malalignment may cause an aberrant distribution of PFJ reaction forces and through this mechanism potentially predisposes to pain and/or structural progression. The presence of patellar translation and complete obliteration of joint space were significantly associated with increased anterior knee pain. The presence of patellar translation was significantly associated with increased difficulty in rising from chair. Joint space narrowing correlates poorly with pain. There is only a weak association between the condition of the articular cartilage and patellofemoral symptoms.

Increased Anteversion

Increased anteversion of the femur persists in some adults and may be the source of patellofemoral dysfunction and pain. Ech off et al. provides the clinical evidence that patients with anterior knee pain unresponsive to conservative management have greater average femoral anteversion than a group of asymptomatic controls. Excessive femoral anteversion can bias the lower extremity internal rotation and may result in the clinical appearance of "squinting patella" and or a toe in gait.

Abnormal Pronation

Abnormal pronation results in a rotatory strain on soft tissue of the lower extremity. Excessive tibia internal rotation caused by abnormal subtalar joint pronation would decrease the Q-angle and the lateral force acting on the patella. To compensate for the lack of tibial external rotation caused by the failure of the foot to resupinate, the femur would have to internally rotate on the tibia such that the tibia was in relative external rotation.

Squatting and Prevalence of Knee OA

In a retrospective study by Liu et al. to find out the association between squatting and the prevalence of knee OA among elders in Beijing, prolong squatting was a strong risk factor for tibiofemoral OA, and a weaker association with patellofemoral OA.

Clinical Features

Patient complains gradual onset of anterior knee pain during activities involving loading the knee in extension due to the pull of the inflamed medial patellar retinaculum and also during activities involving hyperflexion of knee due to stretching of tight lateral patellar retinaculum. Pain is reproduced or aggravated by stair climbing, squatting, sitting with knee bend, etc. activities. Patient may present the history immobilization following any injury or surgery (Fig. 4.2).

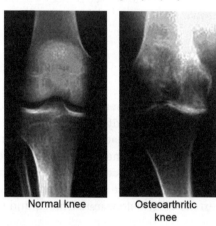

Normal knee   Osteoarthritic knee

Fig. 4.2: X-ray showing osteoarthritic changes.

(*Source:* Victoria BC. How to cope with osteoarthritis and the knee? http://www.victoriawellness.com).

Inspection

Structural malalignment such as genu valgus, femoral anteversion, external tibial torsion, foot pronation in weight bearing, high ridding small patella may be present. Atrophy of vastus medialis obliquus may be present.

Movements

Active knee extension demonstrates excessive lateral tracking of patella at 30–10° of extension. Passive medial gliding is painful and limited; reduced patellar tilting indicates tightness of lateral patellar retinaculum. Weakness of vastus medialis can be elicited by checking resisted quadriceps contraction at 30° of extension and comparing it with the sound side. Clarke's sign may be positive. Obers' test may be positive indicating ITB tightness.

Warmth and tenderness may be present on the back of medial aspect of patella and adductor tubercle, where medial patellar retinaculum is attached.

Management

Strengthening of vastus medialis is very important as it dynamically checks the lateral tracking of patella. Static quadriceps exercise, short arc quadriceps exercise from 30° to 0°, multiangle quadriceps exercise 30°, 10° and 0°, close kinetic knee extension 30° to 0°, SLR are useful. Strong faradic electrical stimulation to VMO also helps for strengthening.

Stretching of the tight lateral structures is very important as it pulls the patella during knee extension. Lateral to medial gliding of patella, medial patellar tilting, etc. help to stretch the tight lateral patellar retinaculum. Taping of patella medially to lift the lateral border of patella may help for normal tracking of patella.

Ultrasound can be applied on the tight lateral patellar retinaculum to improve its extensibility before mobilization and on the medial patellar retinaculum to resolve the chronic inflammation.

Depending on the cause, stretching of ITB, foot wear modification to correct foot deformity and genu valgus, knee orthosis to correct excessive genu valgus, knee orthosis to normally position the patella can be considered.

EXERCISES USED IN THE TREATMENT OF PATELLOFEMORAL PAIN

William Mcmullea et al. December 1990, investigated the effectiveness of selected static and iso kinetic physical therapy rehabilitation program for subjects with a clinical diagnosis of chondromalacia patella. About 29 subjects were screened by orthopedic surgeon and assigned to a control (N = 9), static (N = 11) or isokinetic (N = 9) exercise group. Noncontrol subjects were administered a program of 12 treatments, three times a week, for four weeks. Static exercise program included quadriceps strengthening and hamstring flexibility exercise. Results indicated that the static and isokinetic group demonstrated significant functional improvements over the control group in walking, stair climbing, running, jumping, twisting and overall activity level as well as increased quadriceps strength and hamstring range of motion.

Ingersoll C et al. 1991, demonstrated the effectiveness of electromyography (EMG) biofeedback in specifically recruiting VMO. The training included quadriceps sets and SLR exercises with biofeedback, as well as integrated functional activities of deep knee bends, step ups, and bicycle riding with biofeedback for three weeks. The group that received biofeedback training to decrease VL activity demonstrated an improvement in congruence angle after 3 weeks of training. The control group which received no training showed no significant changes in patella position; whereas the group performing short arc quadriceps femoris exercise with progressive resistance demonstrated a decrease in the congruence angle, even though their quadriceps had improved by 170%. The authors concluded that "terminal extension progressive resistance exercises (in nonweight-bearing) do not produce medial relocation of the patella and may actually predispose individuals to the likelihood of lateral subluxation of the patella.

Michael S, Puniello PT, March 1993, investigated the relationship between ITB tightness and medial glide of the patella in patients with patellofemoral dysfunction. 17 Patients with patellofemoral dysfunction were evaluated. All patients presented with lateral tracking of the patella in knee flexion and extension. Medial glide of the patella was tested manually, and Obers test was performed to test flexibility of ITB. Twelve of seventeen patients exhibited a tight ITB with hypomobility of medial glide of the patella. This study demonstrates a strong relationship between ITB tightness and decreased medial glide of patella.

Gregory M Karst et al. May 1993, did a study to determine whether active exercise accompanying hip adduction with knee extension activate medial components of the quadriceps femoris muscle more than does knee extension alone. The subjects performed quadriceps femoris setting (QS), straight leg raising (SLR), SLR with hip laterally rotated (SLR/LR) and SLR combined with isometric hip adduction (SLR/ADD). EMG activity was recorded from the obliquus (VMO) and longitudinal (VML) portion of the vastus medialis, vastus lateralis (VL), and rectus femoris muscles. Comparison of normalized mean EMG magnitudes revealed that the single joint QF components (VMO, VML and VL) demonstrated significantly greater activity during quadriceps setting (QS) than during any of the three SLR variations and that SLR/LR and SLR/ADD did not elicit greater relative activity of medial QF components than did QS or SLR.

William D Bandy and William P Hanken, July 1993, examined the effect of isometric training of the quadriceps femoris muscles at different joint angles, torque production and EMG activity. Three groups trained with isometric contractions three times per week at a knee flexion angle of 30°, 60°, or 90°. The fourth group which served as a control did not exercise. Measurement was taken before and after 8 weeks of training. Following isometric exercise, increased torque and EMG activity occurred not only at the angle at which subject exercised, but also at angles in the range of motion at which exercise did not occur. Exercise in the lengthened position for the quadriceps femoris (90° of knee flexion) produced increased torque production across all angles measured and appeared to be more effective position for transferring strength and EMG activity to adjacent angles following isometric training as compared with the shorter position of the muscle (30° and 60° of knee flexion).

Stephen M Gryzlo et al. July 1994, described and compared the EMG activity of the rectus femoris, vastus lateralis, vastus medialis obliquus, biceps femoris and semimembranosus with the use of fine wire electrode during five rehabilitative exercise. The exercises were straight leg raising, short arc knee extension, short arc knee extension with hamstring co-contraction, squat, and isometric knee co-contraction.

Conclusion

1. The final 15° of extension during the short-arc knee extension exercise with hamstring co-contraction exercise demonstrated the greatest EMG activity of the vastus medialis obliquus and vastus lateralis than the biceps femoris and semimembranosus.

2. Balanced co-contraction occurred with short arc knee extension with hamstring co-contraction and isometric knee co-contraction exercise at all angles and arcs except during the final 15° of extension in the short arc knee extension with hamstring co-contraction exercise.

3. In squatting the rectus femoris, vastus medialis obliquus, and vastus lateralis were significantly more active than the biceps femoris and semimembranosus during the descending, holding and arising phase.

Kay Cerny et al. August 1995, determined which of selected exercises with and without the feet to move would enhance VMO activity over the VL and whether the use of taping would increase VMO activity. Twenty one subjects were without patellofemoral syndrome and ten were with patellofemoral pain syndrome. Subjects were studied for the normalized, integrated electromyography activity of their VMO, VL, and adductor magnus muscle and VMO/VL ratio using electrodes. Open chain activities were quadriceps femoris muscle setting, knee extension, and isometric holds. All exercises were performed against the resistance of an ankle cuff weight equal to 5% of each subject's body weight to the nearest pound. Closed chain exercises used were (1) walk stance and step-down exercises (2) wall-slide exercises. The results suggest that neither exercises purported to selectively activate VMO activity nor patellar taping improve the VMO/VL ratio over similar exercises.

Snyder–Mackler L et al. 1995, suggested that closed kinetic exercise alone may not provide an adequate stimulus to permit normal function of the knee. Subjects who performed OKC knee extension with high-intensity electrical stimulation demonstrated greater increases in quadriceps femoris muscle torque compared to subjects performing CKC alone.

Deyle et al. 2000, examined the effectiveness of manual therapy and exercise in patients with knee osteoarthritis. A total of 83 subjects (mean age 60 years) were assigned randomly to treatment group or a placebo-control group (subtherapeutic ultrasound) who received treatment 2 times a week for 4 weeks. Outcome measures were distance walked in 6 minutes and the sum of sub scores for pain, stiffness, and function from the Western Ontario and Mcmaster Universities Osteoarthritis Index (WOMAC). The intervention group received a variety of treatments including active range of motion, stretching, strengthening, and manual physical therapy techniques. These techniques were done primarily to the knee, but also to the back, hip, and ankle if limitations were found. Stretching exercises were done for 3 repetitions of 30 seconds and including standing calf stretch, supine hamstring stretch, and prone quadriceps stretch. Active range of motion exercises for knee flexion and extension were performed in long sitting and in sitting during stationary cycling. Strengthening exercises included quadriceps sets (1 set of 10 repetitions with a 6-second hold) and a series of closed chain exercises, including standing terminal knee extension, seated leg press, and step-ups. Resistance or step height was increased as tolerated. Subjects were instructed to perform all exercises at home on the days they were not at physical therapy except the closed chain exercises, and they were instructed to walk daily. The treatment group showed significant improvements in 6 minute walk distance and WOMAC scores at 4 and 8 weeks. The control group did not show any changes. The final measurement taken one year later indicated that WOMAC scores remained lower than baseline values in the exercise group.

NastaKa Sakai et al. 2000, investigated the influence of weakness in the vastus medialis obliquus muscle on patellar tracking on seven human cadaveric knees. They concluded weakness of the vastus medialis caused the patella lateral shift at 0° and 15° of knee flexion.

Quilty B et al. 2003, carried out a RCT of a complex, physical therapy based intervention for knee osteoarthritis with predominant patellofemoral involvement. The participants, who had knee pain and predominant (PFJ OA), were recruited from a large population based study. The physiotherapy intervention comprised of education, quadriceps and functional exercises, and patellar taping delivered by a single physiotherapist in 30-minutes sessions over 10 weeks with advice to continue thereafter. The outcome measures were pain in the worse knee by 100 mm Visual Analogue Score, the disability domain of the WOMAC and quadriceps muscle strength by maximum voluntary contraction. After 10 weeks post-treatment the treatment group had a small decrease in pain and a significant increase in quadriceps strength of the index knee. There was no difference between the two groups at 12 months. A number of limitations to this study existed. First, patients were not reassessed immediately after treatment had ceased but 10 weeks later, thus immediate treatment effects may have been missed. Secondly, patients were not selected on the location/nature of their knee pain. It was possible that some patients may have had symptoms that were not emanating from the knee joint, and thus were unlikely to benefit from such a specific intervention. Thirdly, the patella tape was largely applied by the patients rather than the physiotherapist. Finally, it was not clear how compliant patients were with the exercise program.

Van den Dolder and David L Roberts, 2006, assessed the efficacy of manual therapy for anterior knee pain. Participants were 38 ambulatory care patients with anterior knee pain. The experimental group received six sessions of manual therapy consisting of transverse fiction to the lateral retinaculum as described by Cyriax (1984) conducted both in full extended and fully flexed position, tilt patellofemoral stretches as described by Bruckner et al. 2001, and the application of a sustained medial glide during repeated flexion and extension of the knee. Each session lasting lasted for 15–20 minutes. Outcome measure—pain was measured using the patellofemoral Pain Severity Questionnaire. Activity was measured by having the participants step up and down a 15 cm step, leading with the painful leg as many times as they could in a 60 second period. Effect of intervention: The experimental group reduced their pain by –8 mm (95% CI-17 to 1, P = 0.08) and pain on stairs by –10 mm (95% CI –22 to 2, P = 0.1) compared with the control group.

Hudson Z and Darthuy E, Febuary 2008, proposed that a tight ITB through its attachment of the lateral retinaculum into the patella could cause lateral patellar tracking, patella tilt and compression. Twelve subjects presenting with patellofemoral pain syndrome were compared with twelve matched control subjects. The results from this study show that subjects presenting with patellofemoral pain syndrome do have a tighter ITB.

ELECTRIC STIMULATION USED IN THE STRENGTHENING OF QUADRICEPS

Grimby et al. November 1989, compared contraction forces and discomfort at tolerance stimulation levels during repeated stimulation with high and low frequency stimulation. Low frequency stimulation used rectangular and monophasic impulses with frequencies of 30 Hz–50 Hz corresponding to discharge ratio of motor neurons and resulting in a near tetanized state. It was set at 30 Hz and pulse width 0.3 ms. The other type of stimulation was high (2500 Hz), interrupted sinusoidal pulses with on-off cycles (bursts) of 50 Hz. It was set at a pulse width of 10 μs. Both the stimulation have an initial 2-second ramp of increasing stimulus amplitude. Result showed there were no qualitative differences between the two stimulators in the conceived discomfort. The low–frequency stimulation has a theoretical advantage because of its constant current principle and more constant stimulation effect.

Caggiano et al, July 1990, did a study to see the effects of electrical stimulation over voluntary contraction in strengthening the quadriceps femoris muscles in an aged male population with minimal training. He used biphasic symmetrical square waveform with phase duration ranged from 100 to 113 μs, frequency maintained at 25 pps. Minimal training was defined in this study as 10 contractions per session, with three sessions per week for 4 weeks. Maximum voluntary isometric contraction (MVIC) was measured with a Cybex II dynamometer prior to and following training. The electrical stimulation group trained at an average of 36% of pretest MVIC, the traditional exercise group trained at an average of 42% MVIC.

Results: Average and peak torque values were increased with both modes of training. Both methods of training using a low training load were effective in increasing torque. Electric stimulation has the same potential as traditional exercise to provide improved strength for aged muscles.

Victor AdemokObajulwa, 1991, did a study to see the effect of electric stimulation on quadriceps femoris muscle strength and thigh circumference in healthy young men. He used surged Faradism with square waveform at the largest pulse train of 3 seconds. The current intensity was regulated for maximum tetanic contractions. The maximum contraction possible within the limits of pain was elicited for 3 seconds. This was repeated 10 times with a rest period of 10 seconds between each. The current intensity was gradually increased during each training series until peak tolerance was reached. There were three sessions a week for 10 weeks. Result showed muscle strength and thigh circumference can be significantly increased in healthy young males.

Balogun et al. September 1993, determined the effects of three (20 pps, 45 pps, and 80pps) pulse frequencies, on subjects: (1) Maximum tolerance voltage during stimulation. (2) Poststimulation muscle soreness and (3) Muscle strength following 6 weeks of training.

A high-voltage galvanic stimulation (HVGS) with monophasic (twin-peak pulse) waveform and pulse duration of 65–75 μs was used in this study. Ten maximum contractions were allowed at each training session. Electric stimulation was administered 3 times a week for 6 weeks. The findings revealed that the stimulation used in the study can improve the strength of normal innervated muscles, but none of the three pulse frequencies selected offered any clinical advantage.

Bircan et al. 2002, compared interferential and low frequency currents in healthy subjects in terms of the effects on quadriceps strength and perceived discomfort. They were randomized into three groups.

Group A: This group received electric stimulation with bipolar interferential current with a carrier frequency of 2,500 Hz.

Group B: It received electric stimulation (ES) with low frequency current. The waveform was symmetrical biphasic, with phase duration and frequency of 100 μs and 80 Hz.

Group C: It was control group. The maximum tolerable stimulation intensity was given for 15 minutes, five days a week for three weeks with the knee fully extended in the sitting position. Irrespective of the group assigned, the on-off time of the stimulation was set as 13 seconds on and 50 seconds off. Ramp up time was 2 seconds and ramp down time was 1 seconds. Constant voltage mode was used in both the groups. The current amplitude varied from to 59 mA in group A and 32 mA to 56 mA in group B. Results showed that the MVIC increased for 25% in the low frequency rectangular stimulation group and 13% in the high frequency sinusoidal stimulation.

Callahan et al. June 2004, compared a commercially available electric muscle stimulation regimen with a novel form of stimulation for the rehabilitation of the quadriceps muscle, in patients with patellofemoral pain syndrome. One group (EMPI) received 1 uniform constant frequency component of 35 Hz, asymmetrical biphasic rectangular waveform of maximum amplitude 100 mA, and duty cycle 10:50 delivering 350 impulses per minute with pulse duration 300 μs. The other (EXPER) group received an experimental form of stimulation that contained 5 simultaneously delivered frequency components of 125, 83, 50, 2.5 and 2 Hz with a doublet of pulses (12.5 Hz) at the beginning of each pulse train. Stimulation was applied to the quadriceps muscle of the affected leg for 1 hour daily for 6 weeks at a total of 42 treatments. Result showed patients in both groups showed significant improvements in all outcomes. No difference existed between the stimulation in any outcome.

Durmus D et al. 2007, evaluated the effects of ES program on pain, disability, and quadriceps strength in the patients with knee OA. About 50 women diagnosed as knee OA were randomized into two groups as electric stimulation and biofeedback-assisted isometric exercise. Both of the programs were performed 5 days a week, for duration of 4 weeks. Outcome measure for pain was visual analogue scale pain score and WOMAC. Disability and stiffness were assessed with WOMAC physical function and stiffness score. 1 repetition maximum (RM) and 10 RM were used for measuring quadriceps strength. In addition 50 m walking time and 10 steps stairs climbing up-down time were evaluated. Both groups showed significant improvement in pain, physical function, and stiffness after therapy. There were statistically significant improvement in 50 m walking time and 10 steps stairs climbing up-down time and 1RM and 10RM values indicating the improvement in muscle strength. There were no significant differences between the groups after the therapy. They concluded that ES treatment was as effective as exercise in knee OA and electric stimulation treatment can be suggested especially for the patients who have difficulty in or contraindications to perform an exercise program.

Causes of Primary Osteoarthritis

The exact etiology of osteoarthritis is not known. There are several hypotheses regarding the onset of degenerative joint disease. With aging changes in the cartilage is seen in the nonarticular area of the cartilage, whereas in OA changes occur in those areas of cartilage undergoing most frequent contact doing weight bearing.

Habitual disuse hampers the nourishment of the avascular cartilage, which gets its nutrition from the synovial fluid. Synovial secretion is facilitated by the alternate compression and relaxation of the cartilage, which results from the movements and activities. Therefore prolonged disuse hampers the nourishment of the cartilage resulting in degeneration.

Experiment shows gross changes in rabbit's knee subjected to an impulse load equal to their body weight at a rate of 60 times/minute for 1 hour daily for 30 days. At the sametime many people with heavy body weight, who have done heavy work for most of their lives never experience the symptoms of OA. Therefore, the degree and type of force is more significant to the process of joint wear than the actual total force.

Changes takes place in the region undergoing increase stress with normal activities and changes in subchondral bone will over-time result in changes in articular cartilage and vice versa. Normal attenuation of force applied to a joint is dependent on the elasticity of subchondral bone as well as those of articular cartilage. If stresses are not normally attenuated in one of these tissues, the other will undergo increased stress. With subchondral bone sclerosis, the overlying articular cartilage undergoes increased stress and with fibrocartilage softening subchondral bone undergoes increased stress leading to sclerosis and breaking down of cartilage.

Normally knee joint is loaded at about 10 extension at mid-stance phase of gait cycle. In case of knee flexion deformity, knee remains hyperflexed during the loading phase. In flexion the joint is incongruent. Therefore, the load increases at each loading phase of gait cycle predisposing or precipitating the degeneration. Excessive weight bearing activities with the knee in flexion results in over-loading and predispose to degeneration.

Risk Factors

Reports suggest that OA is associated with different risk factors. Risk factors can be divided into two major categories, systemic factors which are associated with the development of OA and local factors which tend to result in abnormal biomechanical loading of affected joint.

Systemic Risk Factors

Systemic risk factors are the factors thought to contribute to the development of OA by creating a systemic environment where the joint is vulnerable. These factors include ethnicity, age, gender, hormonal factor, genetic factor, bone density, nutritional factor, obesity and other factors which have yet to be identified.

Ethnicity: Anatomic abnormalities that are prevalent in USA are rare in the hip joint of persons of Chinese descent which may indicate the genetic predisposition to developmental abnormalities is a factor in these ethnic variations. However, knee OA is more prevalent in older persons in Beijing than in USA particularly in women. This may be attributable in part to activities thought to be more prevalent in Chinese women such as squatting and manual labor. In USA there are also difference seen some studies in the prevalence and patterns of OA in different ethnic groups. One study showed a higher rate of knee OA in African–American women but not in compared with their Caucasian counterparts however another study showed no difference between these groups. In one study looking at hip OA in men, there was no change in the prevalence in the hip OA between groups but another study showed that African–American men were 35% more likely than white men to have hip OA. Several studies show that African American with hip or knee OA have more severe radiographic features of disease and more frequent bilateral involvement and mobility impairment. These ethnic differences may be related not only to underlying genetic factors but also other variables including variations in body mass index (BMI), nutritional factors and the impact of lifestyle difference and healthcare disparities between populations.

Age: The prevalence and incidence of OA correlates with age. The general condition of radiographic OA in USA population is 1–3% in persons over 55 years of age. In a community-based survey, the incidence and prevalence of OA increased 2-10 fold from 30–65 years of age. The association with age continues until the age of 80 when the curves levels off because they are more sedentary and increase in pain threshold with age. The increase in OA with age is likely a consequence of biologic changes that occur with aging which make it susceptible to disease. These include decrease responsiveness of chondrocytes to growth factors that stimulate repair.

There is also age-related accumulation of advanced glycation end product in cartilage that affects the synthetic and reparative ability of the chondrocytes. In addition, aging is often associated with decreased strength and slower neurologic response attributable in part to a decline in proprioception.

Not only these joint protective mechanisms impaired, but the cartilage also thin increasing shear stress and excessive stress damages the attachment between cartilage and its base thus hastening joint degeneration.

In a Dutch study, by 40 years of age 10–20% of women had evidence of severe radiographic OA in their hand or feet and by age 70 years approximately 75% of women had evidence of radiographic OA in their hands or feet. Schouten et al. reported that patients over 60 years of age had an almost four-fold higher rate of joint space less than those aged 45–49 years.

Gender: Men younger than 50 years have higher incidence of OA than women whereas after age of 50 years women have higher incidence of disease. The difference is also seen in prevalence and it increase with advanced age.

Hip OA is more frequent in men whereas knee, hand and foot OA are more frequent in women. Many factors influence gender difference in incidence and prevalence of OA, including differing occupational history or choice of sports and leisure activities. In addition some developmental abnormalities (Perthes disease, coxa vara, coxa valga) are linked to gender and these conditions are also known to predispose persons to OA as the age progress.

Hormonal status: The evidence regarding the influence of hormonal status on the incidence of OA is mixed. The higher incidence of OA in women who are postmenopausal suggests that estrogen deficiency increase the risk of OA. Estrogen replacement therapy is associated with reduction in the risk of knee and hip OA.

However, high lifetime estrogen exposure correlates with high bone density. Studies on the relationship between high bone density and the development of OA show that high bone mineral density is associated with an increase prevalence of hip, hand and knee OA.

Genetics: Study showed OA has a major genetic component. Primary OA is late onset disease that can be classified as polygenic and multifactorial as environmental factors play a significant role in gene expression. Genetic predisposition to OA could arise from many anatomic structures including cartilage or even from neurosensory input.

About 50% or more of the occurrence of hip joint and hand OA is hereditary. Hereditary of hand OA is high in all joints. Heritability of OA appears to be higher among women than among men for almost all joint. A large scale female twin study showed that a heritability rate of hand and knee OA between 39 and 65% with concordance rate of 0.64 in monozygotic pairs as compared with 0.38 in the dizygotic pairs.

A recent study suggests that generalized radiographic OA is inherited and that the most likely pattern is that of a major Mendelian gene with a residual multifactorial component. The study found that heritability of generalized OA was stronger among female then among men. In some cases, the disease development has been laid to an autosomal dominant mutation in type II procollagen the precursor to type II collagen which is the most prevalent form of collagen in joint cartilage.

Bone density: Osteoporosis and OA have shown to inversely associate in many studies in which individuals with osteoporosis exhibit a lower than expected rate of OA. In additional women with hypertrophic hip OA and osteophyte formation have an 8–12% in which in bone density compared with women without OA. Patients with generalized OA have also been found to have increased bone mass density of the lumber spine.

Nutritional Factors

Theoretically, exposure to dietary antioxidants could have a protective role in the development of OA. The Framingham knee OA Cohort study showed a three-fold reduction is risk for radiographic OA in persons in the middle and highest tertiles of vitamin C intake compared with those whose intake was in the lowest.

The Framingham study demonstrated that the risk for progression of OA was increased three fold for persons in middle and lower tertiles of both vitamin D intake and serum level but there was no association with the risk of new—onset OA.

Obesity: Obesity is associated with high prevalence of knee OA in both genders. Overweight person particularly women develop knee OA more often than people who are not overweight. Obesity is associated with increase in risk of knee OA specifically at patellofemoral compartment, at tibiofemoral compartment and with simultaneous OA at both of these sides.

Increase BMI is also associated with and increase risk of bilateral knee OA. In Framingham study, the BMI measure at entry level into the study predicated the presence of radiographic knee OA 36 years later. Obesity is strong risk factor for subsequent development of bilateral knee OA in those who already have unilateral knee OA.

Studies have shown that obesity is associated with both symptomatic and asymptomatic knee OA and this association is more pronounced in woman. Bilateral hip OA is associated with obesity even when adjusted for age and gender. Some studies have shown that there is an association between obesity and hand OA, with BMI directly proportional to CMC OA in both genders suggesting that obesity may predispose to OA, perhaps via an inflammatory or metabolic intermediary. This means that obesity plays a role not only as local process but systemic as well.

Local Biomechanical Factors

Local biomechanical factors include altered joint biomechanics due to ligament laxity, malalignment, impaired proprioception and muscle weakness, prior joint injury, occupational factors, effect of sports and physical activities and result of developmental abnormalities.

A loss of normal joint biomechanics results in increased joint vulnerability. Individuals who have abnormal joint anatomy or function including disruption incongruity of the articular surface, dysplasia, malalignment, instability, disturbance of innervations of the joint or muscle and inadequate muscle length may have greater risk of OA.

With excessive genu varum, there is compression on the medial aspect of the joint and distraction on the lateral aspect. The weight-bearing shifts to medial compartment. Increased loading overtime will give rise to medial compartment degenerative joint disease. Similarly valgus deformity predisposes to lateral compartment degeneration.

A higher incidence of varus-valgus laxity is seen bilateral in the knee of those with knee OA suggesting that laxity may precede disease development and contribute to the disease process. Impaired proprioception has been seen in patients with OA compared with age match controls, which may also indicate that proprioceptive loss preceded disease development.

The role of mechanical loading in the development of OA is significant. Moderate cyclic joint loading has been shown to be beneficial by enhancing proteoglycans synthesis and making cartilage thicker but continuous compression of the cartilage suppress metabolic activity including collagen and proteoglycans synthesis and causes tissue damage. Joint immobilization has also been shown to be detrimental, reducing cartilage thickness and proteoglycans content. In addition intense exercise or a sudden increase in exercise, particularly in older persons produce catabolic changes in cartilage.

Muscle weakness: Muscle weakness particularly of the quadriceps is often seen in people with OA of knee joint. People with radiographic evidence of OA have been shown to have weaker quadriceps than those without knee OA. Patients with OA who are obese despite have an overall greater quadriceps muscle mass have weaker quadriceps than obese patients without OA. Quadriceps muscle weakness has generally been attributed to disuse atrophy due to pain or altered joint biomechanics.

In a longitudinal study, woman who had no initial radiographic evidence of OA but who did have knee extensor weakness were more likely to develop OA than women with no initial weakness. This suggests that weakness although not necessarily the primary insult to the joint may predispose individuals to the development of OA. Muscle weakness may permit transmission of more loads onto affected OA joints thereby accelerating joint damage.

Hip abductor muscle weakness may result in impaired frontal—plane pelvic control during gait, leading to greater medial compartment loading in people with knee osteoarthritis. Thus, increasing the strength of hip abductor muscle and controlling the pelvis in the frontal plane might reduce joint loading and have disease-modifying effect.[1,2]

OA knee affects hamstring muscle more than the quadriceps muscle. Strengthening the hamstring muscle has been found to enhance the functional ability of deficient knees. The ratio of quadriceps to hamstring muscle strength is important for stability of the knee and for protection from excessive stress.[3]

Joint injuries: OA is associated with a variety of joint injures and damage including fracture of the articular surface, joint dislocation, ligaments and meniscal injuries, etc. Loss of articular cartilage may result from single injury i.e. chondral or osteochondral fracture or from repetitive injuries, that cause splits in the articular surface.

Studies of both human and animal models convincingly demonstrate that a loss of ACL integrity, damage to the meniscus and meniscectomy lead to knee OA. Follow-up studies of patients with cruciate rupture have reported cartilage loss even in young patients and the risk rises with advanced age. Major injuries that alter mechanical function or joint alignment may also predispose individuals to OA at other sites.

Factors that are associated with altered joint shape lead to local stress on the cartilage and predispose individuals to cartilage loss and early diseases. Articular surface incongruity can also increase local contact stress and predispose the joint to accelerated development of OA. Other risk factors for development traumatic OA include high body mass, high level of activities and residual joint instability and malalignment.

Occupation: The development of OA is associated with repetitive joint loading in daily activities as life-long normal daily activities and regular recreational activities have not been shown to increase the risk of joint degeneration. The repetitive loading of normal joint can exceed the joint tolerance and leads to degeneration of joint structure. Occupational activities in which there is repetitive use of particular joint groups include Jackhammer operator, shipyard worker, coal miners, farmers and pneumatic drill operators lead to OA in joints exposed to repetitive occupational use. Women whose jobs involved repetitive pincer grip motion had a higher rate of distal interphalangeal joint OA than other women whose job did not involve repetitive grasp. Studies demonstrated a significant increase in knee OA in men and women who engage in jobs that are associated with high physical demands, i.e. miner, dockworker, concrete worker and shipyard workers as compared with clerical and office staff.

Jobs requiring kneeling and squatting also predispose individuals to knee OA and jobs with heavy lifting can lead to hip and knee OA. Hip OA occur two to eight times more frequently than expected among agricultural laborers, may be due to regular lifting of very heavy loads and walking ever rough ground.

Sports and physical activities: Certain types of sporting activities have been associated with increased risk of OA. The runners under 50 years who run more than 20 miles per week have higher risk of developing OA. The risk of OA increases with joint damage, ligament damage or meniscal injury sustained during sports activities.

High intensity, acute, direct joint impact as a result of contact with other players or equipment can increase the risk of OA in affected joint. Torsional loading also seems to be associated with joint degeneration, i.e. elbows of throwing athlete. Early diagnosis and treatment of sports-related injuries with a goal of maintaining joint surface integrity should help decrease the subsequent risk of developing OA at the injured joint.

Primary osteoarthritis is distinguished from secondary by the elimination of predisposing factors and relevant pre-existing diseases of the knee such as involving tibial plateau and/or femoral condyles, instability after ligamentous injury, postinflammatory states—TB, septic arthritis, etc. and deformity—genu valgum, genu varum, foot or hip problems, following meniscectomy or patellectomy, etc. Primary OA is considered to be a result of aging.

Pathogenesis

Osteoarthritis involves all the structures that form the synovial joint, which include articular cartilage, subchondral bone, synovial membrane, ligament, joint capsule and muscle those cross the knee joint (Fig. 4.3).

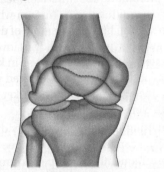 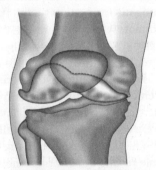

Healthy knee joint   Hypertrophy and spurring of bone and erosion of cartilage

Fig. 4.3: Osteoarthritis of knee.

Osteoarthritis/degenerative joint disease is characterized by progressive degenerative changes in articular cartilage and sub-chondral bone. The tissue changes may be of a compensatory hypertrophic nature such as bony proliferation that typically occurs at the margin and the subchondral bone or capsular fibrosis. Cartilage is designed to withstand a great amount of wear and fear, composed of cells, collagen fibers and mucopolysaccharides. The first change is loss of mucopolysaccharides with the loss of elasticity and reduced ability to protect the cells by absorbing shock, leading to further damage. Initial fibrillation and irregularities of the superficial zone of the articular cartilage develop and extend into the transitional zone. The focal regions of cartilage loss with cleft and fissure develop along with changes in the deepest layer of cartilage, the calcified cartilage layer. When loss of cartilage is full thickness the bone get exposed. On cellular level, there is an imbalance between the destructive and reparative or synthesis process of the articular cartilage. The mechanism responsible for progressive loss of cartilage in OA includes alteration of the cartilage matrix, decline of the chondrocytic synthetic response and progressive loss of cartilage.

Histological studies localized areas of softening in which the cartilage becomes irregular (fibrillation). Clefts develop and in time extend down to, and penetrate, subchondral bone with the formation of cysts.

The degenerated detached articular cartilage fragment needs to be removed from the joint. So there develops mild-to-moderate inflammatory process and the synovium gets inflamed. As inflammatory process subside the synovial fluid become thick and glue the synovial tissue and ligaments. Adhesion formation limits joint mobility. In chronic stage of disease fibrosis and thickening of capsule and intracapsular structures lead to stiffness. Fibrosis or thickening of the outer fibrous layer of the joint capsule is caused by an increased production of collagen and by a decrease in the ground substance. It can occur in chronic irritation or inflammation caused by imbalanced stresses moving through the joint. A tight, fibrotic capsule results in abnormal movement between the joint surfaces, leading to excessive compression in certain areas of the cartilage and to accelerated degeneration of the joint.

As bone get involved in disease process, there is formation of new extra bone on trabeculae in the subchondral bone gradually it leads to subchondral sclerosis, formation of cyst like bone cavities and development of osteophytes. Development of osteophyte due to changes in articular cartilage develop around the periphery of the joint and also along insertions of the joint capsule. Subchondral bone alterations are thought to be result of abnormal osteoblast function. Microfracture of the highly elastic cancellous subchondral bone may occur due to excessive load, leading to fracture of subchondral trabeculae which healed by callous formation and remodeling. The remodeled trabeculae are stiffer than normal so reduce the shock absorbing ability of the subchondral bone.

With the progressive degeneration of articular cartilage and subchondral bone, the joint space reduces resulting in capsular laxity, hypermobility and instability. With the destruction of the smooth articular surface, there will be crepitus during the movement from increased friction between the articulating surfaces.

With pain and decrease willingness to move, contracture eventually develops in portions of the capsule and overlying muscles so that as disease progress, movement becomes more limited. Decrease use of the joint lead to muscle atrophy with concomitant loss of joint protection.

Osteoarthritis pain develops mainly from synovium, joint capsule, periarticular tender points and subchondral bone as all of these structures have large number of group IV nociceptors.[8] In osteoarthritis, there may be sclerosis and marginal proliferation of subchondral bone that leads to the development of osteophytes which are responsible for stimulating nociceptors situated in the densely innervated periosteum and in the walls of blood vessels that permeate bone. Group IV nociceptors in the synovium and capsule become mechanically stimulated when the pressure in the joint increases. They become chemically stimulated when inflammation induced tissue damage leads to the liberation of nociceptor sensitizing substance such as bradykinin, prostaglandin, serotonin, histamine and neuropeptides. In addition pain may develop as a result of the calcium crystal-induced inflammatory changed (Dieppe et al. 1976).[8]

Tender points are found commonly in anteromedial aspect of upper part of tibia, where the lower part of the collateral ligament and superficial to this the tendon of the sartorius, gracilis and semitendinosus muscle insert into the tibia. Tenderness in this site may also be due to inflammation of the anserine bursa situated between the ligament and these tendons. Tenderness may also be located along the edges of the patella, particularly along its lateral upper border. Posterior tender points are frequently found to be present in the popliteal fossa, particularly at the center of it and on its insertion.[8] These tender points activity give rise to pain at the back of the knee joint during the course of running or walking, particularly when going down hills or downstairs.

Clinical Features

Insidious onset of pain following weight-bearing activity such as walking, stair climbing, getting up from sitting, etc. Later as low-grade inflammation develops, the patient complains of morning pain and stiffness, which subsides following movements and activity and returns back with increase intensity following activity due to fatigue. Then pain is felt during activity continuously.

At the onset the pain following activity is due to fatigue. As the inflammation set in pain becomes continuous. Pain during activity is because of stretching of the tight capsule. With the erosion of subchondral bone which is highly pain sensitive pain becomes continuous. Once joint instability develop due to gross destruction of the articular cartilage, strain on the periarticular capsule-ligamentous structures gives rise to pain. Impingement of soft tissue structure by the marginal osteophyte also give rise to localized inflammation and pain. Synovial nipping may give rise to pain.

Observation: Walks with limping and finds difficulty in squatting, getting up from sitting, stair climbing, etc.

Inspection: Atrophy of thigh, more of vastus medialis.

Deformity: Knee flexion deformity due to capsular contracture and varus due to destruction of medial compartment of tibiofemoral joint.

Movements: Active and passive knee movements limited in capsular pattern, i.e. flexion beyond 90° and terminal extension beyond 20° is limited. Crepitus present. Resisted isometric knee flexion-extension is painless.

Joint play: Passive patellar movements are limited. Tibial glidings over femur are also limited. Internal rotation of tibia is limited and painful due to tightness of posteromedial capsular tightness.

Palpation: Warmth, swelling and joint line tenderness present in joint effusion stage. Localized pain may be present due to irritation of the soft tissue by the osteophyte.

Management

Avoid weight-bearing activities with knee bend such as prolonged walking, stair climbing, prolonged sitting with knee bend, squatting, etc. to reduce joint loading. Reduce body weight. Associated causative factors such as pronated foot, leg length discrepancy, etc. can be managed by modified foot wear. Knee orthosis realign the medio-lateral malalignment, i.e. varus so that medial compartment can be deloaded and further degeneration can be minimized. One can use walking stick to reduce transmission of body weight through the joint.

- ❑ Strengthening of the quadriceps and hamstrings
- ❑ Strengthening of abductor muscle[1,2] (Figs. 4.4 and 4.5)
- ❑ In the presence of joint effusion high voltage pulsed galvanic stimulation, interferential therapy, strong faradic electrical stimulation or TENS can be used for pain relief
- ❑ Low–level laser can also be used for pain relief[4]
- ❑ Whole body vibration reduces pain and improves function[5,6]
- ❑ Hydrotherapy improves strength and function[7]
- ❑ Dry needling on popliteus muscle is also helpful in reducing pain (but there is no literature).

When knee movements are limited in capsular pattern traction, capsular stretching, soft tissue massage, mobilization techniques,

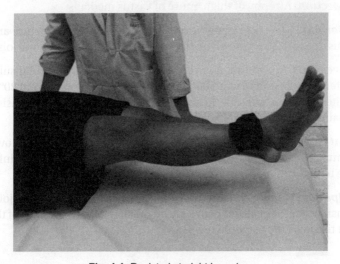

Fig. 4.4: Resisted straight leg raise.

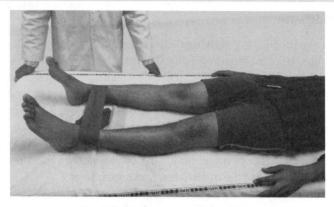

Fig. 4.5: Hip abductors strengthening.

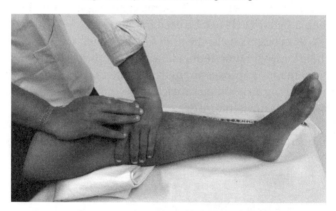

Fig. 4.6: Superior to inferior glide of patella.

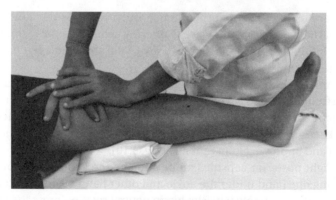

Fig. 4.7: Inferior to superior glide of patella.

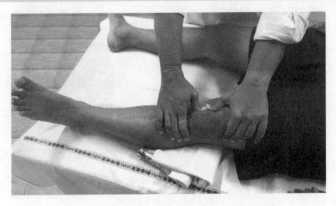

Fig. 4.8: Medial to lateral glide of patella.

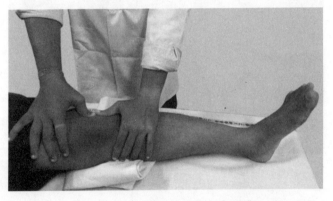

Fig. 4.9: Lateral to medial glide of patella.

etc. are useful to stretch the tight capsule, which is the source of pain. Ultrasound or short wave diathermy before manual technique is helpful to improve the extensibility of the short collagen tissues (Figs. 4.6 to 4.9).

Ankle traction with pillow under the ankle, hip in neutral rotation and fixation of the lower thigh by a belt stretches the short periarticular structures. Soft tissue massage around the patella and on the back of the knee, more over the posteromedial aspect is effective in reducing pain and improving joint mobility (Fig. 4.10).

Tight posterior capsule can be stretched in supine position by placing one hand under the ankle and other hand over the anterior aspect of lower thigh; with the hip in neutral rotation press the knee

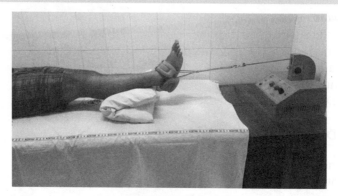

Fig. 4.10: Ankle traction.

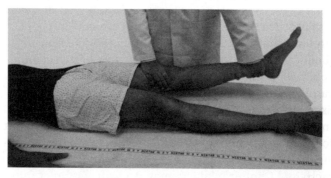

Fig. 4.11: Posterior capsule stretching.

down while raising the heel up. In prone position with pillow under the lower thigh and ankle out of the bed, fix the thigh by one hand and hold above the ankle by the other hand, rotate the leg inward and extend the knee with traction so that patient will experience discomfort on the back of the knee (Fig. 4.11).

In prone position with pillow under the lower thigh, leg and foot out of the bed, fix the thigh by one hand and leg is stabilized between Therapist's legs. Rotate the leg inward, apply traction to the leg and move the proximal tibia backward to forward with the other hand. It mobilizes the knee to restore full knee extension.

Stretching of hamstrings, TA, hip adductors, external rotators is also essential to relief pain and reorientation of the joint.

Gait re-education, activity modification such as use commode instead of Indian mode of toileting, sit on a correct height chair to avoid excessive knee bending, avoid prolonged standing, stand with the affected limb forward, avoid stair climbing, while climbing progress with the sound limb and while descending progress with the affected, use the hand railing to transfer some body weight through it.

Diet control and regular exercises reduces over weight.

CHONDROMALACIA PATELLAE

Chondromalacia patellae (Fig. 4.12) is the softening articular cartilage of patella in an otherwise fit person. Females are more affected than males with 3:1. Age of onset is between 15 to 18 years. This condition is commonly seen in joggers and long distance runners, referred as runner's knee. The exact cause is not known. It typically occurs in physically active people aged <40 years, it also affects people of all activity levels and ages.[8] Bilateral involvement is more than unilateral. Frequently persistent over years without getting worsen or improved. Immobilization following trauma or surgery reduces the stress over the cartilage precipitating the degeneration.

Excessive lateral tracking of patella results in compression of odd medial facet of the patella. It may results from osseous factors, static ligamentous imbalance, dynamic muscular imbalance or biomechanical factors related to the proximal or distal joints, overactivity.[9] Chondromalacia may occur from direct injury or biochemical changes. Its etiology is still unclear but the process is thought to be due to trauma to superficial chondrocytes resulting in a proteolytic enzymic breakdown of the matrix.[10] Knee pain from the irritation of this degenerated cartilage during activities often referred to as patellofemoral syndrome, anterior knee pain, runner's knee, and formerly chondromalacia patellae.[8]

Chondromalacia is a degenerative process thought to be due to overloading of articular cartilage lining patella. Compression of the articular cartilage results in deficiency of nutrition and malacia. In stage-I, localized softening and inflammation of articular cartilage occurs. There is fibrillation of the articular cartilage of patella in stage II. Gradually, the fissure widens and deepens to take the appearance of crab meat, stage III. Finally, full thickness cartilage defect extends up to the subchondral bone the degenerated cartilage gets detached and the subchondral bone becomes exposed. There develops synovitis to remove the degenerated articular cartilage.

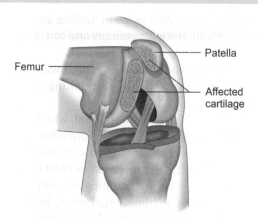

Fig. 4.12: Chondromalacia patella.
(*Source:* http://www.ncbi.nlm.nih.gov/pubmedhealth/PMH0001488/).

Clinical Features

Insidious onset of vague aching or soreness on the retropatellar area, which aggravates with prolonged knee bending such as sitting, stair climbing, kneeling, squatting, running, etc. Knee movements are associated in crepitus. Mild swelling of knee may be present. Stiffness experienced following sitting. Patient often complains of giving way or locking.

Effusion and atrophy of quadriceps, more of VMO are present. Resisted knee extension is painful. Decreased knee extensor strength is a common finding,[10] hypermobility of patella present and apprehension test may be positive. Tenderness over medial articulating surface of patella and medial femoral condyle is present. Compression of patella against femoral condyle is painful.

X-rays are normal and arthroscopy is diagnostic.

Clinical classification of patellofemoral pain and dysfunction:

1. Patellofemoral instability
2. Patellofemoral pain, with malalignment but no episode of instability
3. Patellofemoral pain without malalignment.[11]

Management

Acute stage: Rest with crepe bandage, static quadriceps exercise, active ankle foot exercise, straight leg raising in all directions.

Subacute stage: Pulsed SWD helps in healing and relaxed passive movement to maintain the joint mobility and soft tissue extensibility are given.

Gradually partial weight-bearing crutch walking, progressive strengthening, endurance, passive stretching and mobilization exercises are given.

Strengthening of VMO is very important, which can be achieved by short arc knee extension exercise, static quadriceps exercise, SLR, progressive resisted short arc knee extension exercise and resisted SLR, etc. exercises. Electrical stimulation to VMO is also useful.

Mini squat, cycling, climbing, running, etc. can be added as pain allowed. Stretching of hamstrings, quadriceps, lateral retinaculum, TFL, ITB, TA help in restoring normal knee joint motion. Patellar mobilization, soft tissue mobilization,[12] tapping and orthosis help in normal tracking of patella. Modification of activities to reduce patellofemoral compressive force is essential. Intervention aimed at controlling hip and pelvic motion (proximal stability) and ankle/foot motion (distal stability) should be considered when treating patient with PFA.[12]

If it does not respond to conservative treatment corticosteroid injection can be tried. If it fails arthrotomy may be tried otherwise patellectomy is the last choice.

OSTEOCHONDRITIS DISSECANS

Osteochondritis dissecans (Fig. 4.13) is the localized avascular necrosis of medial femoral condyle. The exact cause is not known. Males are more affected than females and occurs during the 2nd decade.

It is assumed that medial femoral condyle gets injured or impinged against the spine of tibia resulting in thrombosis of the end artery supplying the joint. So there develops avascular necrosis of the articular cartilage. The necrosed cartilage becomes soft and gets detached, remains inside the joint as loose body. The gap in the articular cartilage is filled up by fibrocartilage. To remove the loose body out of the joint, there develops synovitis and joint effusion.

Patient with osteochondritis dissecans demonstrate a high rate of sports activities and/or trauma prior to the onset of symptom.[13]

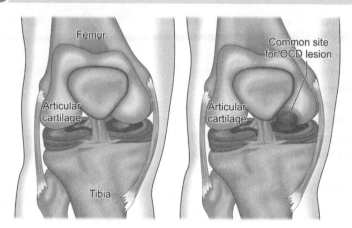

Fig. 4.13: Osteochondritis dissecans.

(*Source:* American Academy of orthopaedic Surgeons. http://orthoinfo.aaos.org/ topic.cfm?topic=A00610).

Clinical Features

Patient complains of pain on exertion and compensatory lateral rotation of tibia during gait.[14] History of locking with limitation of joint range of motion in noncapsular pattern. As effusion develops, pain worsens and joint range of motion gets limited in capsular pattern.

Reproduction of pain by internal rotation of tibia during knee extension between 90 to 30° of flexion and then relieving that pain by externally rotating the tibia.[14]

Management

Before dislodgement drilling into the underlying healthy bone to improve circulation. After dislodgement surgical removal of the loose body.

OVERUSE INJURY

Injury to knee may not be always related to trauma. Repetitive nature of activity, e.g. running may produce an injury overtime. The relative risk of overuse injury was significantly higher among persons with the most valgus knee.[15]

Cumulative stress overtime may exceed the reparative capability of the involved tissue giving rise to chronic inflammation and pain. Continued activities in the presence of pain leads to pattern of abnormal use or disuse of the part resulting in the development of stiffness and weakness.

Female are more affected than male because of structural and biomechanical difference (Excessive Q-angle and genu recurvatum are more common in women than men) may place added stress on the knee, increasing the likelihood of an overuse injury.[16]

OSGOOD-SCHLATTER'S DISEASE

Osgood-Schlatter's disease (Fig. 4.14) was described in 1903 by Osgood, USA and Schlatter, Germany. Tibial tubercle is an extension of proximal tibial epiphysis and serves as the point of attachment for quadriceps. Excessive traction on tibial tubercle due to overactivity or inefficiency of extensor mechanism in growing bone, i.e. before apophysis unites lead to overgrowth of the tibial tubercle. This overuse syndrome occurs in late childhood or early adolescence (10–15 ages of age) in basketball, soccer, and gymnastics, etc. athletes, where running, jumping, sprinting, etc. activities, which demand excessive knee extensor activity, are the precipitating factors. The regular practice of sports in the pubertal phase and the shortening of the

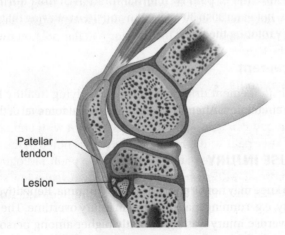

Patellar
tendon

Lesion

Fig. 4.14: Osgood-Schlatter's disease.
(*Source:* http://www.islandorthotics.org).

rectus femoris muscle were the main factors associated to the presence of OS syndrome in the students.[17]

Few findings indicate a strong association between Osgood-Schlatter disease and patella alta. This increase in patellar height would require an increase in the force needed from the quadriceps to achieve full extension. This mechanism could be responsible for the apophyseal lesion.[18]

Clinical Features

Tenderness and swelling are present over tibial tubercle. Pain aggravates with vigorous physical activity, kneeling and crawling, relieved with rest. Pain is reproduced with resisted knee extension and terminal range of passive knee flexion. Flexibility of quadriceps, hamstrings and TA is reduced. Quadriceps atrophy is present and occasionally quadriceps lag may be present.

Differential Diagnosis

Sinding–Larsen–Johansson Syndrome

Sinding-Larsen-Johansson (SLJ) syndrome is a traction apophysitis of the inferior patellar pole. The pathology is analogous to OSS except for the involvement of the inferior pole of the patella. Children present between ages 10 and 12 years with complaints of knee pain localized to the inferior patella. Slight separation and elongation or calcification is noted radiographically at the inferior patellar pole on the lateral view of the knee.[19]

Hoffa's Syndrome

The infrapatellar fat pad is a richly innervated tissue. Any injury to the fat pad can cause pain. Patients present with complaints of anterior knee pain, and maximal tenderness is noted in the anterior joint line lateral to the patellar tendon. The plain radiographs are usually normal. MRI scans characteristically reveal a low signal on all sequences within the fat pad due to fibrin, hemosiderin and/or calcification.[20]

Synovial Plica Injury

Synovial plicas are normal synovial folds within the knee joint. They are remnants from embryological development of the knee. The mediopatellar or infrapatellar plica connects the lower pole of the patella to the intercondylar notch. Trauma and repetitive motion cause thickening, fibrosis and hemorrhage in this plica, giving rise to anterior knee pain. It can be diagnosed by MRI, which shows a curvilinear high T2 signal intensity within Hoffa's fat pad in the line of infrapatellar plica.[21]

Tibial Tubercle Fracture

Tibial tubercle fracture usually occurs in boys between the ages of 12 and 17 years. The mechanism of injury is violent contraction of the quadriceps or forceful flexion of the knee when the quadriceps is contracted. Patients present with complaint of pain, local swelling, knee effusion and an inability to actively extend the knee.[22]

Management

In acute stage ice compression provides symptom relief. Avoid all precipitating activities such as running, jumping, kneeling, knee bending, strenuous lower limb exercises, etc. Cycling and swimming are good substitute for exercise. Simple patellar support, knee sleeve may help in pain relief and is recommended in case of severe pain with difficulties in activities of daily living. Cylindrical plaster cast immobilization may be considered for those who do not comply with the advice to take rest.

Stretching and strengthening exercises to maintain balance between anterior and posterior structures is important. Stretching of quadriceps, hamstrings and TA; and strengthening of quadriceps and dorsiflexors reduces strain on tibial tubercle. Electrical stimulation to quadriceps to overcome extension lag and resisted SLR are useful.

Persistent pain following closure of proximal tibial epiphysis may be due to presence of loose ossicles, which requires excision.[23,24] One can return back to activity once bony union has occurred.

When patients fail extensive nonoperative management, surgery to remove the symptomatic ossicle should be offered after skeletal maturity. When this is the case, the addition of tubercleplasty should be performed.[18]

Soft Plastazote orthotics or heel cups are useful as most common associated problem is foot pronation.[26]

PATELLAR TENDONITIS (JUMPER'S KNEE)

It is a chronic overuse injury of patellar tendon causing pain at the inferior pole of the patella.[27] As its name implies, it frequently occurs in athletes who must jump excessively in their sport, e.g. volleyball, basketball, etc. The prevalence is particularly high in athletes.[28,29] Among elite volleyball and basketball players a prevalence over 40% has been described (Fig. 4.15).[30]

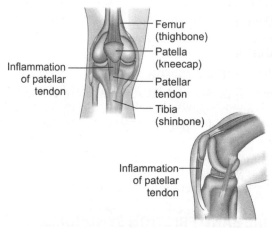

Fig. 4.15: Jumper's knee.
(*Source:* Patellar tendon injury. http://www.summitmedicalgroup.com).

The etiology of patellar tendinopathy is not completely understood, but repetitive overload is thought to be an important factor.[31,32] It may also occur in individuals who perform excessive lifting of weight in the quadriceps.

Overuse results in chronic inflammatory changes of the quadriceps tendon giving rise to pain, tenderness and swelling. Continued activities lead to progressive attrition of the tendon and rupture of weaken tendon. Tight hamstrings and TA are the aggravating factors.

Clinical Features

Pain aggravates in activities that load the quadriceps including jumping, lifting weights, running downhill, etc.

Patellar tendonitis (Jumper's knee) is characterized by pain during resisted knee extension. Passive knee flexion may be painful and limited. Extension lag may be present.

On palpation, localized tenderness over patellar tendon and swelling may be present.

Management

Avoidance of all the activities those precipitate the condition. Ultrasound helps in resolution of chronic inflammation. Transverse friction massage breaks the adhesion, realigns the collages tissues, and improves its strength and extensibility. Stretching of quadriceps, hamstrings and TA are helpful.

For reducing pain isometric exercise in mid-range as tolerated, reduce loading on the area and activity modification is necessary. Strength progression is done by isotonic exercises of knee, progressive resistance exercise program, endurance training. Progression can be done by increase speed of muscle contraction and lowering the number of repetition, plyometric exercises, etc.[33]

Recent researchers have shown the positive effect of extra-corporeal shockwave therapy for treatment of patellar tendinitis.[34]

ILIOTIBIAL BAND FRICTION SYNDROME

With flexion and extension of knee ITB moves backward and forward overlateral epicondyle of femur. Repetitive flexion/extension may irritate it proximally at its origin on the ilium, distally at the insertion on anterolateral portion of proximal tibia, initiating inflammatory process. When painful irritation occurs proximally over the greater trochanter, it is referred as snapping hip syndrome and when it manifests distally over the lateral femoral epicondyle it is referred as runner's knee (Fig. 4.16).

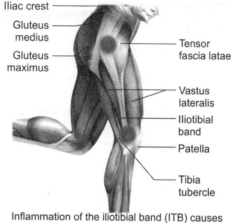

Iliac crest

Gluteus medius

Gluteus maximus

Tensor fascia latae

Vastus lateralis

Iliotibial band

Patella

Tibia tubercle

Inflammation of the iliotibial band (ITB) causes outer knee pain and possible pain in the hip.

Fig. 4.16: Iliotibial band friction syndrome.

Several etiologies have been proposed for ITB syndrome including friction of ITB against lateral femoral epicondyle, compression of fat, synovial cyst at knee and connective tissue deep to the IT band and chronic inflammation of IT band bursa. Mechanical irritation is more pronounced in individual with tight ITB, prominent lateral epicondyle, varus alignment of knee, leg length discrepancy (short leg), etc.

Extrinsic factors such as sudden increase in mileage of running, running on uneven ground (limb on downhill side), running in shoes with excessive lateral heel wear, running on hard surface, etc. also predispose or precipitate the condition.

According to a research the development of iliotibial band syndrome is related to increased peak hip adduction and knee internal rotation. These combined motions may increase iliotibial band strain causing it to compress against the lateral femoral condyle.[35]

It frequently occurs in distance running, downhill skiing, circuit training, weight lifting, jumping sports, cycling, etc. Activities requiring repeated knee flexion and extension.

Clinical Features

Complains of pain on lateral side of knee, which aggravates with initiation of running activity and improves with activities, again return back with increase intensity following activity. Pain also aggravates with ascending or descending stairs.

Snapping of ITB present at about 30°–40° of knee flexion/extension. Pain is reproduced on involved limb in knee flex about 30°-40° which brings the ITB in contact in lateral epicondyle of femur. Localized tenderness present over the lateral femoral epicondyle and occasionally swelling may be present.

Ober's test often becomes positive indicating ITB tightness and Noble compression test is also positive.

Management

Avoid the precipitating activities, such as downhill running, running on uneven ground, prolonged running, etc.

In the acute stage cryotherapy is applied and in the subacute phase ultrasound/phonophoresis with salicylate cream or 10% hydrocortisone may be applied locally for pain relief. Moist heat may be used prior to stretching followed by icing.

Deep transverse friction massage (DTFM) followed by stretching of tight IT band and TFL or myofascial release and trigger point release may be given. According to research most effective method of IT band stretching is with arm extended overhead.[36]

In runners recovery phase, focuses on series of exercises to improve hip abductor strength and integrated movement patterns and final return running phase is begun with another day program, starting with easy sprints and avoidance of hill training with gradual increase in frequency and intensity.[37]

Footwear compensation is necessary in case of limb length discrepancy and footwear modification in case of foot deformity such as medial heel wedge in case of pronated foot, lateral heel wedge in case of supinated foot or genu varum can be prescribed. Soft footwears are preferred.

PREPATELLAR BURSITIS

Prepatellar bursa interposed between the skin that overlies the patella and patella itself, eliminating friction between skin and patella (Fig. 4.17). Its location makes it susceptible to direct trauma due to fall on knee giving rise to acute bursitis. Chronic bursitis often referred as housemaid's knee results from repeated direct blows due to prolonged quadruped posture as in case of plumbers, carpet layers, wrestlers, football players, etc.

Other causes of prepatellar bursitis is infection by bacteria (e.g. *Mycobacterium marinum, Staphylococcus aureus*).[38,39] Noninfectious etiologies of bursitis include trauma; gout; sarcoid; idiopathic calcification; and calcinosis, Raynaud phenomenon, esophageal dysmotility, sclerodactyly, and telangiectasia (ie, CREST) syndrome.

Acute inflammation with local extra-articular swelling is present in acute bursitis, which can be managed by rest, ice, compression, elevation and anti-inflammatory drug. Aspiration followed by compression of more painful bursa not responding to conservative treatment may be required. After 48–72 hours, once acute inflammation subsides gentle range of motion (ROM) exercise without pain and static quadriceps exercise can be initiated. Gradually eccentric, concentric and progressive resisted strengthening exercises and stretching of the adjacent structures can be given. Prophylactic padding should be given while returning to activity.

In chronic bursitis, both the layers of bursa become thicken, distended and adherent restricting the movements. Insidious onset of anterior knee pain. Pain with joint ROM is a typical except for discomfort at extreme flexion, which compresses the inflamed bursa. It can be managed by heat therapy such as ultrasound or shortwave diathermy, which increases the circulation and soften the bursal layers. Progressive strengthening exercises, stretching of the adjacent structures and prophylactic padding should be given before returning to activity.

Excision of bursa may be considered in case of recurrence.

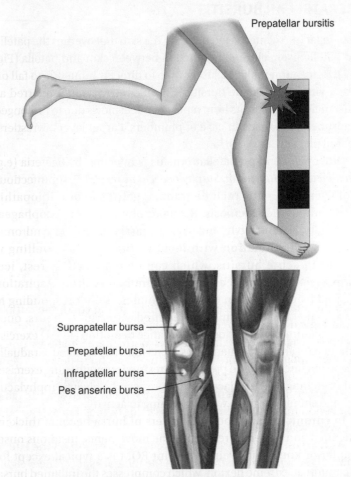

Prepatellar bursitis

Suprapatellar bursa
Prepatellar bursa
Infrapatellar bursa
Pes anserine bursa

Fig. 4.17: Prepatellar bursitis.

(*Source:* Prepatellar Bursitis or Beat Knee or Carpet Layer's Knee. http://www.epainassist.com/sports-injuries/).

GENU VALGUM

Knock-knees (genu valgum) is an angular deformity at the knee where the apex of the deformity points toward the midline (Fig. 4.18).

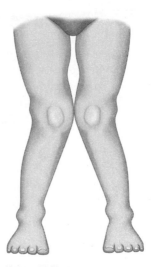

Fig. 4.18: Genu valgum.

In the adults the leg should be straight. In the child, the normal physiological development of knee is from varum to straight, to valgum and again to straight. In the newborn, there is genu varum. It becomes straight at about 18–19 months of age, there develops genu valgus at about 3–4 years of age and again becomes straight at about 6 years of age. Lower extremity alignment goes through a predictable progression from varus (bow-legs) to valgus (knock-knees) over the first seven years of life.[40]

With excessive genu valgum, there is compression on the lateral aspect of the joint and distraction on the medial aspect. The weight-bearing shifts to lateral compartment. Increased loading overtime will give rise to lateral compartment degenerative joint disease. There will be excessive tensile stress over the medial collateral ligament and capsule resulting in ML laxity. Increased Q-angle will give rise to lateral patellar tracking dysfunction and anterior knee pain. There develop secondary foot pronation and foot pain.

Causes: Static genu valgum may develop secondary to gravitational force or foot pronation. Dynamic genu valgum develop due to IT band tightness or tight vastus lateralis. Asymmetrical epiphyseal growth, i.e. under growth due to damage of lateral upper tibial and/or lower femoral epiphysis or overgrowth due to acute inflammation of medial upper tibial and/or lower femoral epiphysis gives rise to genu valgum. It is very common in rickets.

Causes of genu valgum include physiologic valgus, post-traumatic, systemic/metabolic conditions, skeletal dysplasias and neoplasms. Flat feet and external tibial torsion may accompany physiologic valgus and can accentuate its appearance.[41] Children younger than 10 years of age who sustain a fracture of the proximal tibia are at risk for developing valgus deformity secondary to selective medial physeal overgrowth in response to the fracture or the healing response (Cozen fracture).[42] Knock-knees also may be caused by many systemic/metabolic medical problems (e.g. rickets, mucopolysaccharidosis), skeletal dysplasia (e.g. multiple epiphyseal dysplasia, pseudoachondroplasia), and neoplasms (e.g. multiple hereditary exostoses).[41,43]

Clinical Features

Clinically genu valgum can be classified into ligamentous, osseous and compensatory. Ligamentous genu valgum deformity is more in weight-bearing than that in nonweight-bearing. Osseous genu valgum deformity remains same both in weight bearing and nonweight-bearing. Knee bending test demonstrate whether the abnormality is in tibial or femoral component. On bending the knee if the deformity disappears then the defects is in femoral component, if the deformity persists then the defect is in tibial component. Compensatory genu valgum deformity develops to equalize the opposite short limb.

Degrees of genu valgum can be measured by goniometer. Measure the intermalleolar distance by measure tape with the condyles of knee in contact with each other. Both the measurements should be taken both in weight-bearing (standing) and nonweight-bearing (supine lying) positions.

Management

Ligamentous genu valgum deformity can be managed by knee orthosis, genu valgum secondary to foot pronation can be corrected by foot wear modification. Osseous deformity can be managed by knee orthosis during the growing age, if not corrected surgery will be required. Compensatory genu valgum requires foot wear compensation to equalize the limb length.

Closed wedge osteotomy from the medial side or open wedge osteotomy from the lateral side of upper tibia or lower femur depending on whether the tibia or femur is involved. Closed wedge osteotomy gives rise to shortening whereas open wedge osteotomy gives rise to lengthening of the limb post operatively. Postoperatively the osteotomy site may be fixed by internal fixation and plaster cast immobilization is given for 6–8 weeks.

Stapling of the overgrowing epiphysis during the growing phase arrests asymmetrical growth and also corrects the deformity.[44]

GENU VARUM

Bow-legs (genu varum) is an angular deformity at the knee where the apex of the deformity points away from the midline (Fig. 4.19). It is a condition in which the knees of an affected individual are wide apart, while the ankles and feet are together when the person stands up.

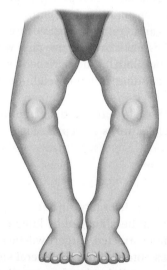

Fig. 4.19: Genu varum.

With excessive genu varum, there is compression on the medial aspect of the joint and distraction on the lateral aspect. The weight-bearing shifts to medial compartment. Increased loading overtime will give rise to medial compartment degenerative joint disease. There will be excessive tensile stress over the lateral collateral ligament and capsule. There develop secondary foot supination.

Osseous genu varum develops commonly in rickets and osteo-arthritis. Asymmetrical epiphyseal growth, i.e. under growth due to damage of medial upper tibial and/or lower femoral epiphysis or overgrowth due to acute inflammation of lateral upper tibial and/or lower femoral epiphysis gives rise to genu varum.

Clinical Features

Clinically, genu varum can be classified into ligamentous, osseous and compensatory. Ligamentous genu varum deformity is more in weight-bearing than that in nonweight-bearing. Osseous genu varum deformity remains same both in weight-bearing and nonweight bearing. Knee bending test demonstrate whether the abnormality is in tibial or femoral component. Compensatory genu varum deformity develops to equalize the opposite short limb.

Degrees of genu varum can be measured by goniometer. Measure the intercondylar distance by measure tape with the malleoli in contact with each other. Both the measurements should be taken both in weight-bearing (standing) and nonweight-bearing (supine lying) positions.

Radiographs, though optional as a rule, may be needed to differentiate physiologic varus from pathologic conditions that call for treatment.[45]

Management

Ligamentous genu varum deformity can be managed by knee orthosis, osseous deformity can be managed by knee orthosis during the growing age and if not corrected, surgery will be required.

Closed wedge osteotomy from the lateral side or open wedge osteotomy from the medial side of upper tibia or lower femur depending on whether the tibia or femur is involved. Closed wedge osteotomy gives rise to shortening whereas open wedge osteotomy gives rise to lengthening of the limb postoperatively. Postoperatively the osteotomy site may be fixed by internal fixation and plaster cast immobilization is given for 6–8 weeks.[46]

Stapling of the overgrowing epiphysis during the growing phase also corrects the deformity.

In genu varum due to osteoarthritis of the knee in very advanced cases, the joints are replaced called total knee replacement surgeries. If only inner half of the joint is replaced it is called unicondylar knee replacement and if all the three chambers of the joints are damaged, then the entire knee joint is replaced and is called the total knee replacement.[47]

KNEE FLEXION DEFORMITY

A flexion deformity of the knee is the inability to fully straighten the knee. In people with a flexion deformity either flexion or extension or both are reduced.

Normally peak weight-bearing force is transmitted at mid-stance or loading phase of the gait cycle, during which the knee remains about 10° flexion, near closed pack position where tibiofemoral contact area is more; so the load is less. In case of knee flexion deformity one has to load the joint in more flexed position, where tibiofemoral contact area is reduced than normal; so the loading will be increased. It will predispose or precipitate degeneration of tibiofemoral joint. That is the reason why full extension must be restored before restoration of flexion range of motion and weight bearing in bend knee should be discouraged.

Early changes are shortening of stride gait, reduced popliteal angle and a flexed position of the knee at the initiation of the stand phase and throughout gait cycle. Changes which appear later are severe contracture of knee and hip and patella alta.[48]

Knee flexion deformity develops due to muscle imbalance by the overactivity of the hamstrings. Knee flexion is a comfortable position; knee flexion without extension in prolonged recumbent persons develops knee flexion deformity due to adoptive shortening of posterior knee structures. Painful knee arthritis, effusion associated with spasm of hamstrings may lead to knee flexion deformity.

Management

Moist heat or paraffin wax can be used prior to stretching and mobilization of the knee to supple the overlying skin, improve extensibility of the short soft tissue structure around the joint and relief pain.

Sustained stretching of hamstrings and TA may be given. Joint mobilization techniques include patellar mobilization in supine, external rotation of tibia and posterior to anterior gliding of tibia over femur in prone.[49]

Patient must do active free exercises to maintain or improve the extension range of motion. In prone lying with the foot out of the bed and pillow under the knee to relief pressure on the patella, swing the leg into extension. Check rotation of the thigh. In supine lying or in long sitting with pillow under the heel press the knee down, rotation of the thigh must be checked. Static quadriceps exercise should be done as many times as possible.

In painful knee flexion deformity skin or tibial skeletal traction may be used. Use sand bag or pillow to prevent rotation of the thigh. One must do static quadriceps exercise as many times as he can do. Manipulation under anesthesia followed by plaster cylinder and serial correction may be considered in case of resistant knee flexion deformity.[50] Deformity more than 40 may require soft tissue release after a period of traction followed by traction and plaster immobilization. Deformity more than 40 may require corrective supracondylar osteotomy of femur and internal fixation after a period of traction followed by plaster immobilization.[51]

GENU RECURVATUM

Static genu recurvatum is associated with genu valgum/varum deformity. Ligamentous laxity, asymmetrical epiphyseal growth, i.e. under growth of anterior upper tibial and/or lower femoral epiphysis or over growth of posterior tibial and/or lower femoral epiphysis, compensatory to equalize with the opposite short leg etc. are various causes of genu recurvatum (Fig. 4.20).

In case genu recurvatum line of gravity falls anterior to knee joint and creates an extension moment, which stabilizes the knee in weight-bearing in persons with quadriceps weakness. In case foot equines, line of gravity falls anterior to knee joint creating an extension moment and pushes the knee back into genu recurvatum. It may develop due to muscle imbalance as in case of hemiplegics due to spasticity of quadriceps. According to Kendall et al. "postural faults that persist can give rise to discomfort, pain, or disability".[52]

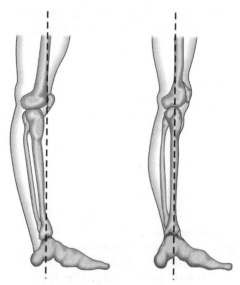

Fig. 4.20: Genu recurvatum.
(*Source:* Knee injuries. http://www.iocdme.com/kneeinjuries.htm).

Management

Management depends on the cause. Genu recurvatum due to ligamentous laxity during childhood may be managed by knee orthosis, a brace that attempts to prevent hyperextension of the knee and makes it stable during the growth period. Genu recurvatum due to quadriceps weakness may require orthosis, till muscle balance is restored. Genu recurvatum in spastic can be managed by relaxation of quadriceps, strengthening of it, stretching of plantar-flexion, strengthening of dorsiflexors, and correction of pelvis retraction.

Rehabilitation of the individual with genu recurvatum should focus on biomechanical correction, proprioception training, muscle control, gait training, and functional activities.[53] Knee control during gait can be taught in conjunction with the exercises. Noyes et al. recommend that the patient maintain knee flexion of 5" throughout the stance phase of gait.[54]

REFERENCES

1. Elizabeth A, et al. Effect of a home program of hip abductor exercise on knee joint loading, strength, function, and pain in people with knee osteoartheritis: a clinical trial. PTJ. 2010; 90(6):895-904.
2. Powers CM. The influence of abnormal hip mechanics on knee injury: a biomechanical perspective, level of evidence; aetiology/therapy, level 5. J Orthop Phys Ther. 2010;40(2);42-51.
3. Ahmed H Al-Johani, et al. Comparative study of hamstring and quadriceps strengthening treatments in the management of knee osteoartheritis. J Phys Ther Sci. 2014;26(6):817-20.
4. Hegedus B, et al. The Effect of low-level laser in knee osteoartheritis: A double blind, randomized, placebo-controlled trial. Photomed Laser Surg. 2009;27(4):577-84.
5. Zafar H, et al. Therapeutic effects of whole body vibration training in knee osteoarthritis: a systemic reviews and meta-analysis. ArchPhys Med Rehabil. 2015.
6. Park YG, et al. Therapeutic effects of whole body vibration on chronic knee osteoarthritis. Healthways Medical Groups. 2015.
7. Foley A, et al. Does hydrotherapy improve strength and physical function in patients with osteoarthritis –a RCT comparing gym based and a hydrotherapy based strengthening programme. Ann Rheum Dis. 2003; 62(12):1162-7.
8. Crossley KM, et al. Patellofemoral pain. Br J Sports Med. 2016 50:247-50.
9. Thomee R, et al. Patellofemoral pain syndrome. Sports Medicine.1999; 28:245-62.
10. Macmull S, et al. The role of autologous chondrocytes implementation in the treatment of symptomatic chondromalacia patellae. International Orthopaedics. 2012;36:1371-7.
11. Holmes SW, Clancy WG. Clinical classification of patellofemoral pain and dysfunction. Journal of Orthopaedic & Sports Physical Therapy.1998; 28:299-306.
12. Powers CM. The influence of altered lower-extremity kinematics on patellofemoral joint dysfunction: a theoretical perspective. Journal of Orthopaedic & Sports Physical Therapy. 2003;33(11):639-46.
13. Bruns J, Klima H. Osteochondrities dissecans of the knee and sports.1993;7(2):68-72.
14. Conrad JM, et al. Osteochondrities dissecans. Am J Sports Med. 2003; 5:777-8.

15. Cowan DN, Jones BH, et al. Lower limb morphology and risk of overuse injury among male infantry trainees. Medicine and Science in Sports and Exercise.1996;28(8):945-52.
16. Devan MR, et al. A prospective study of overuse knee injuries among female athletes with muscle imbalances and structural abnormalities. Journal of Atheletic Training. 2004; 39(3):263-7.
17. de Lucena GL,dos Santos Gomes C, Guerra RO. Prevalence and associated factors of Osgood-Schlatter syndrome in a population-based sample of Brazilian adolescents. Am J Sports Med. 2011; 39(2);415-20.
18. Aparicio, G, Abril JC, Calvo E, Alvarez L. Radiologic study of patellar height in Osgood-Schlatter Disease.Journal of Pediatric Orthopaedics: January/February 1997;17(1);63-6. Journal of Pediatric Orthopaedics: October/November 2007; 27(7):844-7.
19. Medlar RC, Lyne ED. Sinding–Larsen–Johansson disease. Its etiology and natural history. J Bone Joint Surg Am. 1978;60:1113-6.
20. Jacobson JA, Lenchik L, Ruhoy MK, et al. MR imaging of the infrapatellar fatpad of Hoffa. Radiographics. 1997;17:675-91.
21. Peace KA, Lee JC, Healy J. Imaging the infrapatellar tendon in the elite athlete. Clin Radiol. 2006; 61:570-8.
22. Watson-Jones R. Injuries of the knee (revised by Trickley EL). In: Wilson JN,(Ed). Fractures and joint injuries. Vol 2, 5th edition. Edinburgh: Churchill Livingston; 1976;pp.1047-50.
23. Flowers MJ, Bhadreshwar DR. Tibial tuberosity excision for symptomatic Osgood–Schlatter disease. J Pediatr Orthop. 1995;15:292-7.
24. Ferciot CF. Surgical management of anterior tibial epiphysis. Clin Orthop.1955; 5:204-6.
25. Ferciot CF. Surgical management of anterior tibial epiphysis. Clin Orthop.1955; 5:204-6.
26. Lyle JM, Lloyd M. Prevention and management of calcaneal apophysitis in Children: an overuse syndrome.Journal of Pediatric Orthopaedics. 1987.
27. Blazina ME , Kerlan RK , Jobe FW. Jumper's knee. Orthop Clin North Am. 1973;4:665-78.
28. Lian OB, Engebretsen L, Bahr R. Prevalence of jumper's knee among elite athletes from different sports: a cross sectional study. Am J Sports Med. 2005:33:561-7.
29. Zwerver J, Bredeweg SW. Prevalence of jumper's knee among non-elite athletes from three different sports. Abstract book of the XXIX FIMS World Congress of Sports Medicine, Beijing, 2006:273.
30. Bahr R, Fossant B, Løken S, et al. Surgical treatment compared with eccentric training for patellar tendinopathy (Jumper's Knee). A randomized, controlled trial. J Bone Joint Surg Am. 2006;88:1689-98.
31. Alfredson H. The chronic painful achilles and patellar tendon: research on basic biology and treatment. Scan J Med Sci Sports. 2005;15:252-9.

32. Kannus P. Etiology and pathophysiology of chronic tendon disorders in sports. Scand J Med Sci Sports.1997;7:78-85.
33. Rudavsky A, Cook J .Physiotherapy management of patellar tendinopathy. Journal of Physiotherapy. 2014; 60:122-9.
34. Leeuwen, et al. Extracorporeal shockware therapy for patellar tendinopathy: a review of the literature. Br J Sports Med.2009; 43:163-8.
35. Noehren B. Prospective study of the biomechanical factors associated with iliotibial band syndrome. 2007. ASB Clinical Biomechanics Award Winner 2006; 22(9):951-6.
36. Fredericson M. Quantitative analysis of the relative effectiveness of iliotibial and stretches. Archieve of Physical Medicine and Rehabilitation. 2002;83:589-92.
37. Fredericson M, Weir A, et al. Practical management of iliotibial band friction syndrome in runners. Clinical Journal of Sport Medicine. 2006;16:261-8.
38. George Ho, et al. Septic bursitis in the prepatellar and olecranon bursae. Ann Intern Med. 1978;89(1): 21-7.
39. Winter FE, et al. Prepatellar caused by Mycobacterium marinum. J Bone Joint Surg Am.1965;47(2):375-9.
40. Salenius P, Vankka E. The development of the tibiofemoral angle in children. J Bone Joint Surg Am. 1975; 57:259.
41. Kling TF Jr. Angular deformities of the lower limbs in children. Orthop Clin North Am. 1987;18:513.
42. Ogden JA, Ogden DA, Pugh L, et al. Tibia valga after proximal metaphyseal fractures in childhood: a normal biologic response. J Pediatr Orthop. 1995; 15:489.
43. Barrett IR, Papadimitriou DG. Skeletal disorders in children with renal failure. J Pediatr Orthop. 1996;16:264.
44. Stevens PM, et al. Physeal stapling for idiopathic genu valgum. Journal of Pediatric Orthopaedics. 1999; 19: 645.
45. Levine AM, Drennan JC. Physiological bowing and tibia vara. The metaphyseal-diaphyseal angle in the measurement of bowleg deformities. J Bone Joint Surg Am. 1982;64(8):1158-63.
46. Murphy SB. Tibial osteotomy for genu varum. Indications, preoperative planning and technique. The Orthopedic Clinics of North America. 1994;25(3):477-82.
47. Neyret P, et al. Total knee replacement in severe genu varum deformity. Interact Surg. 2008;3:6-12.
48. Wheeless' Textbook of Orthopaedics (secondary).
49. Steffen T. Low-load, prolonged stretch in the treatment of knee flexion contractures in nursing home residents. Phys Ther. 1995;75:886-97.
50. Suksathien R. A new static progressive splint for treatment of knee and elbow flexion contractures. 2010;93(7):799-804.

51. De Morasis Fiho MC, Neves DL, et al. Treatment of fixed knee flexion deformity and crouch gait using distal femur extension osteotomy in cerebral palsy. J Child Orthop. 2008;2(1):37-43.
52. Kendall FP, McCreary EK, Provance PG. Muscles: testing and function, 4th edition. Baltimore: Williams and Wilkins; 1993.
53. Rubinstein RA, Shelbourne KD, VanMeter CD, McCarroll IR, Rettig AC, Gloyeske RL. Effect on knee stability if full hyperextension is restored immediately after autogenous bone-patellar tendon bone anterior cruciate ligament reconstruction. Am J Sports Med.1995; 23(3):365-8.
54. Noyes FR, Dunworth LA, Andriacchi TP, Andrews M, Hewett TE. Knee hyperextension gait abnormalities in unstable knees. Am J Sports Med.1996; 24:35-45.

Chapter 5

Fractures and Dislocations

INJURY TO EXTENSOR MECHANISM

Isolated tearing of individual muscle belly of the extensor apparatus does not cause great trouble, as the other muscles can compensate for the damage. However, extensive adhesions or fibrosis can cause a disabling loss of flexion of the knee. The rupturing of the extensor apparatus that matters is the rupture of any part of the fibrous structure lying across the front of the knee joint, containing the patella. Rupture of the apparatus may or may not include patella.

Fracture Patella

Clean cut transverse fracture without separation is caused by direct blow, e.g. falling on the knee in which patella gets fractured without displacement or damage to medial and lateral expansions.

Transverse fracture with separation is caused by indirect violence of forced flexion against resistance, e.g. stumbling, knee is being flexed by body weight while quadriceps violently contacting to save the individual from falling; in which there is disruption with separation across front of the joint of variable degree. Following fracture the proximal fragment gets retracted upward and the gap between the fracture segments is filled up with hematoma. If it is left like that healing occurs by fibrous union with lengthening of the tendon and permanent loss of active knee extension.

Comminuted fracture: Comminuted fracture patella is caused by direct blow. Patella gets crushed against the femoral condyles. Quadriceps tendon is not ruptured, so full active knee extension is possible.

Management

In the transverse fracture without separation power of extensors is not lost. It is managed by aspiration followed by plaster cast or posterior slab immobilization for 2–4 weeks. No surgery is required. Walking is allowed immediately once the plaster becomes dry. Static quadriceps exercise and nonweight-bearing mobilization exercises can be started after a few days.

Transverse fracture with separation should be managed by open reduction internal fixation by screw or tension wire followed by plaster cast immobilization for 2/3 weeks. After plaster removal nonweight-bearing range of motion exercises and after 6 weeks partial weight-bearing crutch walking is allowed.

In case comminuted fracture, if displacement is minimal and articular surface is smooth, posterior slab immobilization is given for 2/3 weeks. Weight-bearing is allowed immediately. The findings suggest that neuromuscular electrical stimulation (NMES) in conjunction with traditional quadriceps strengthening exercises may have had the ability to improve quadriceps strength in these individual with comminuted patellar fracture and ORIF surgery.[1]

In case of displacement with damage to articular cartilage, restoration of perfect joint surface is not possible. It is therefore managed by excision of patella and quadriceps tendon is sutured firmly followed by immobilization for 3–4 weeks. Immediately after patellectomy, active ankle and foot movements should be encouraged. Static quadriceps exercise can be started after day 1. Active/active assisted straight leg raise (SLR) can be initiated once plaster becomes dry. Nonweight-bearing active knee range of motion exercise starts after plaster removal. Partial weight-bearing crutch walking can be allowed after 4/5 weeks. Passive knee mobilization and progressive quadriceps strengthening exercises can be given after 6 weeks. Full weight-bearing can be allowed once adequate quadriceps strength is regained and patient returns back to activities after 8–12 weeks.

Rupture at upper margin of patella: Avulsion of rectus femoris occurs in elderly. Palpable gap present above the patella, unfortunately it is missed.

Recent injury requires repair by suturing tendon to patella followed by plaster cylinder immobilization for 3–4 weeks. Postoperative treatment protocols in the literature range from early mobilization with full weight-bearing to cast immobilization for up to 12 weeks.[2]

Avulsion of ligamentum patellae from patella: Patella is retracted up by the pull of quadriceps and active extension is lost. If the rupture is not repaired by early of suture, hematoma below the lower pole of patella undergoes ossification either fuses with patella or scattered myositis ossificans traumatica will be formed, depending on whether the joint is immobilized or not.

It should be managed by stitching ligamentum patella securely to the inferior pole of patella followed by immobilization for 4/6 weeks. A complete functional restitution after surgical treatment at least with regard to the activities of daily living, can be achieved in most cases, especially if performed during the first few days after injury.[3]

Avulsion of ligamentum patellae from tibial tubercle: More violent injury, e.g. landed into sitting position in high jump, may cause avulsion of the tendon of insertion of quadriceps from tibial tubercle in younger age group, below 18 years of age, before fusion of the tubercle.

In adults it is rare. Forceful manipulation of knee under anesthesia may result in crack of the tubercle or slightly separated tubercle.

In younger persons avulsed tibial tubercle is fixed by ORIF by screw followed by plaster immobilisation for 8/10 weeks. In adults power of active knee extension is not lost. so no immobilization is required. It is managed like soft tissue injury; active nonweight-bearing knee flexion is practiced. But forceful flexion has to be avoided.

LATERAL DISLOCATION OF PATELLA

Acute Dislocation

Cause—Trauma

1. A common mechanism of patellar subluxation/dislocation is a rotational force involving external rotation of tibia in relationship to the femur, with strong quadriceps contraction; the patella undergoes a sudden shift in the lateral direction resulting in subluxation/dislocation, e.g. cutting away from the affected side.

2. A second mechanism for subluxation/dislocation is a severe abduction force on an extended knee while the foot is fixed on the ground and quadriceps contracted.

Quadriceps contraction places the patella in a high riding position and it lies where the trochlear surface of the femur is the shallowest.

Clinically, patient finds difficulty in moving the knee unless it is reduced. Later the knee swells from an effusion of fluid, which may be blood stained, if the medial capsule is torn, local tenderness present anteromedially from strain or rupture of capsule. There is no significant difference between conservative and operative treatment for patients after first-time traumatic patellar dislocation.[4]

Recurrent Dislocation

Incidence is more common in female due to increased Q-angle.

Generally occurs during adolescence, thereafter dislocation tends to recur with increasing ease, usually when the knee is being straightened from flexion or semiflexed position.

Causes

1. Increased Q-angle, genu valgum
2. Shallow intercondylar groove because of underdeveloped lateral femoral condyle.
3. High riding patella (small patella)
4. Generalized congenital joint laxity (laxity of medial joint capsule).
   Because of abnormal joint mechanism, there is risk of early degenerative joint disease.

Habitual Dislocation

Habitual dislocation is uncommon, occurs at a much younger age—often in early childhood.

Cause

Shortening of quadriceps, particularly vastus lateralis, often resulting from intramuscular injection in infancy.

1. Abnormal fibrous and tethering the vastus lateralis to iliotibial band (ITB), so patella is pulled laterally out of the groove each time knee is flexed.

Management

Acute stage

1. *Initial rehabilitative phase:* Rest with compression bandage and elevation, ice therapy 20 minutes 5/6 times per day for 48 hours.
   - For resolution of effusion and pain relief, Faradic stimulation, high voltage galvanic stimulation, interferential therapy, transcutaneous electrical nerve stimulation (TENS) or biofeedback can be used
   - Walking with a pair of crutches is allowed as the initial discomfort subsides, weaned from crutches as soon as possible
   - For range of motion (ROM), knee flexion in high sitting as pain allows and for flexibility, slow and sustained stretching of hamstrings, TA, ITB, etc. for at least 30 seconds should be given
   - For muscle strength, static quadriceps exercise, multiangle isometric quadriceps exercise, SLR for hip flexion, abduction, adduction and extension are given.
2. *Intermediate rehabilitative phase:* Intermediate rehabilitative phase starts when swelling and pain subside and joint range of motion (JROM) improved.
   - For strengthening without aggravating pain or swelling, short arc knee extension from 90° to 45° can be initiated
   - ROM, flexibility and isometric exercises are continued
   - Swimming, cycling, etc. can be given to improve the endurance.
3. *Advanced rehabilitative phase:* Advanced rehabilitative phase starts when swelling and pain subside and JROM is within normal limit.
   - Progressive strengthening, endurance, ROM and flexibility exercises continued. Full flexion should be regained
   - Partial weight-bearing exercises can be initiated
   - Gradually increase duration, distance and intensity of walking.
4. *Final phase:* Final rehabilitative phase starts when isokinetic evaluation shows quadriceps and hamstrings strength 70–80% of sound side.
   Running program can be started—light jogging, running, running with turning, running in figure of '8' path, circle running, running with sharp cut and gradually return to sports once isokinetic evaluation shows quadriceps and hamstrings strength 85–90% of sound side.

Elastic knee sleeve with a ½" felt cut in the shape of 'C' along the lateral border of patella can be used.

Surgery for Recurrent Dislocation of Patella

Static Realignment Procedure

1. *Lateral retinacular release*—cutting of all the laterally based structures such as lateral patellofemoral ligament, lateral synovium and a portion of proximal vastus lateralis, so that the patella can be everted approximately 45°. Otherwise adhering tissue band of synovial tether must be cut after release, the patella should easily sublux medially. Arthroscopic lateral release successfully treats recurrent patellar dislocations in adolescents, influences functional recovery and improves knee function.[5]

   Following surgery compressive dressing is applied to prevent postoperative hemarthrosis.
   - Early mobilization, i.e. medialization of patella should be given to prevent occurrence of excessive scarring and fibrosis
   - Active ankle foot toes movements and static quadriceps exercise should be done immediately, electrical stimulation to vastus medialis can be given
   - Active and passive knee ROM exercises, patellar mobilization in all directions, SLR in all directions can be initiated after 72 hours
   - Crutch walking is allowed once pain and swelling subside.
   - After 3rd week progressive strengthening, ROM, swimming, static cycling, etc. are given.
   - Full weight-bearing is allowed after 7 to 8 weeks provided there is no pain or swelling and X-rays shows healing
   - Then advanced rehabilitative phase begins, where progressive strengthening, endurance, flexibility, balance training, etc. are given, so that patient returns back to activities between 2 to 6 months.

2. *Distal realignment procedure:* Medialization of patellar tendon by elevating the tibial tuberosity is done. The tendon with the bony attachment is reattached to a new bed and fixed by screw. The aim of the surgery is to changes Q-angle. Under correction may lead to lateral subluxation and over correction may result in medial

subluxation. So correction must be planned, tested properly by moving the patella medially and laterally at the time of surgery until the surgeon is satisfied in the tracking of the patella on the operating table.

- Bone to bone healing becomes stronger. 6 weeks plaster cylinder cast immobilization is given
- Immediate postoperatively active ankle foot toes movements and static quadriceps exercise should be done and electrical stimulation to vastus medialis can be given
- Patellar mobilization can be started between 3–5 days. SLR can be started once the plaster becomes dry and then partial weight-bearing crutch gait can be initiated
- If postoperatively immobilization is given by posterior splint/ hinged cast brace active/passive ROM can be initiated as soon as it is tolerated by the patient.
- Full weight-bearing is allowed by 7–8 weeks provided there is no pain or swelling and X-rays shows healing.
- Then advanced rehabilitative phase begins, where progressive strengthening, endurance, flexibility, balance training, etc. are given, so that patient returns back to activities after 6 months.

Dynamic Realignment Procedure

1. Vastus medialis is cut from its attachment on patella and is transferred distally to a new attachment on patella so that the resting length of it increases; thereby the force exerted by it also increases to correct patellar alignment and tracking. The length must be adjusted properly, otherwise over lengthening will result in patellar rotation which may exacerbate a pre-existing patellofemoral chondrosis and under lengthening will result less dynamics force to correct the subluxation/dislocation.

Postoperatively 3–6 weeks immobilization by plaster cast cylinder or posterior splint and compressive dressing (RJ bandage) or hinged cast brace. Immediate postoperatively active ankle foot toes movements and static quadriceps exercise should be done. Early partial weight-bearing crutch gait can be initiated once the plaster becomes dry.

After 3 weeks, active ROM exercise, SLR can be started and full weight-bearing can start after 6 weeks. Return to activities after 6 months.

2. Tube realignment procedure to avoid prolonged immobilization and thereby atrophy. The aim of surgery is to change of overall vector pull of quadriceps mechanism, i.e. Q-angle. Lateral half of ligamentum patellae is cut, passed underneath the medial half and reattached to patellar retinaculum medially.

Soft tissue to soft tissue anastomosis requires 2–3 weeks immobilization till wound heals. RJ dressing is applied to control postoperative swelling. After stitch removal active knee movements can be started and after 6 weeks activities are allowed.

A systemic review of 4 meta-analysis by Erickson et al. found that operative treatment of acute patellar dislocations may result in lower scale of recurrent dislocations than nonoperative treatment, but did not improve functional improvement.[6]

Dr John Fulkerson, MD, 2007, according to him making a decision regarding proximal or distal realignment in a patient with recurrent patella instability is challenging. Some surgeons favor performing proximal realignment exclusively by medial patellofemoral ligament tendon graft reconstruction or full medial imbrication after lateral release. Other orthopedic surgeons almost always move the tibial tubercle medially in the patient with recurrent patella instability.[7]

FRACTURE SHAFT OF FEMUR

Fracture shaft of femur is usually sustained by severe violence like road accidents. Fracture may occur by direct force due to road traffic accidents or by indirect force due to twisting and bending. It may occur at any site, i.e. in upper, middle and lower thirds and may be transverse, oblique, spiral or comminuted in nature depending upon force.

Following fracture proximal fragment is flexed abducted and externally rotated due to pull of the muscles attached to it and the distal fragment is adducted due to pull of adductors. There is overriding of fragments by muscular pull and shortening. Malalignment results in faulty use of the limb and strain on the joints. Loss of forward bending of shaft may increase the strain in knee.

Diagnosis can be made from the history of violence followed by classic signs of fractures like pain, swelling, warmth, abnormal mobility, deformity—axial deviation, shortening. Radiological examination of femur in 2 planes confirms the diagnosis.

Fracture displacements are reduced either by manual traction, distraction table or with distracter. Fracture segments are preferably reduced with distracter. Dummy nail with handle are used for joystick reduction maneuvers, i.e. the proximal fragment is realigned with distal fragment by slight adduction or abduction movements.

Two Schanz screws for distraction may be placed in same planes or different planes and inserted to proximal and distal fragments and distraction force applied by manipulating the external rod connected to the Schanz screws.

Butcher et al. reported that only 72% of people treated for lower extremity fractures at level-I trauma facilities were able to return to work at 12 months after injury and that 82% were able to return to work at 30 months after injury and these results indicated that after 1 year, the chances of returning to work declined. Although authors reported that all measurements of impairments were obtained by physical therapists, no standard rehabilitation program was described.[8]

For plating skin incision is placed on lateral side of thigh between greater trochanter and lateral femoral condyle. Fascia latae is splitted and vastus lateralis is retracted along the intermuscular septum down to linea aspera. For plating with less invasive exposure 3–5 cm long incision is placed anterolaterally. After reduction of fragments, the submuscular route for plate fixation along the shaft of femur is done with elevator through that incision.

Choice of Implants

About 95° angled blade with anatomical reduction and tight fixation is choice of treatment for simple fracture. Dynamic condylar screws with bridging plates are used for complex fracture. Proximal femoral nail introduced from tip of greater trochanter gives a stable construct for subtrochanteric fracture. For complex multifragmented diaphyseal fracture of femur, the locked intramedullary nail—reamed, unreamed, or cannulated is the choice of implant. If for any reason nailing cannot be performed, a bridge plate (broad DCP 4.5 or broad LC-DCP 4.5) can be used–preferably after indirect reduction and using the tunneling technique.

Skin or pin traction using Thomas's splint with person knee flexion attachment to allow knee flexion and extension through 60° without interfering fracture union.

Complications

Damage to the quadriceps may occur by the sharp edges of the fracture segments, which undergo fibrosis and adhesion formation leading to limitation of knee flexion. Quadriceps also develops atrophy and weakness.

Joint effusion of the knee may result in adhesion formation and knee stiffness.

Prolonged immobilization for the conservative management may give rise to respiratory and circulatory complications. Foot drop due to TA tightness and clawing of toes may also result.

During immobilization for 12 weeks, immediately after surgery active ankle foot and toes movements helps to prevent development of circulatory complications, maintain foot posture. Deep breathing exercises, forced expiratory techniques help to prevent respiratory complications.

Static quadriceps exercise to prevent atrophy and adhesion, maintain mobility of patella, prevent development of effusion, etc. can be started once the initial reaction subsides, usually after 4/5 days. Static hamstrings exercise helps in maintaining the extensibility of quadriceps.

Bilateral upper limb exercises, crutch exercises, exercises for the other lower limb prevent disuse atrophy and help in strengthening.

Following immobilization: Nonweight-bearing crutch walking, nonweight-bearing mobility and strengthening exercises should be given for 1 month. Then partial weight bearing crutch walking, vigorous mobilization and progressive strengthening exercises should be given. Full weight-bearing is allowed once the fracture is healed properly.

To avoid prolonged immobilization, functional cast brace can be given after 4–6 weeks, once the fracture is glued adequately.

Internal fixation, K-nailing can be done by closed method with the aid of image intensifier and guided wire or open reduction internal fixation.

Depending on the rigidity of fixation, patient may be allowed to move freely on bed followed by weight-bearing after a few days in case of rigid fixation or may be rested with traction or Thomas splint for 3–4 weeks followed by partial weight-bearing by crutches. Sometimes cast bracing is given for walking.

SUPRACONDYLAR FRACTURE FEMUR

Of all femoral fractures, approximately 4–7% are distal femur fractures (Kolmert, 1982). Supracondylar fracture femur occurs about 9 cm above the articular surface, in adults at any age due to high energy trauma or in elderly with low energy trauma due to osteoporosis. Approximately, 85% of these fractures occur in patients over 50 years of age (Shewring, 1992).

Patients are typically unable to ambulate. They have severe pain, swelling and varying amount of deformity above the knee. Patients may present with vascular and neurological compromise. In young, continuous traction immobilization and in elderly to prevent the complications of prolonged immobilization, open reduction internal fixation and early mobilization is preferred. The small supracondylar fragment is nearly always displaced backwards and held flexed by the unopposed action of gastrocnemius resulting in genu recurvatum. Popliteal artery may be damaged/compressed by the sharp margin of the lower fragment. A thorough neurovascular examination is essential along with examination of spine and extremity. There may be varus angulation by the pull of adductors and shortening.

Injury to the quadriceps muscle fibers by the sharp margin of the upper fragment lead to fibrosis and gross adhesion, limiting knee flexion range.

AP, lateral and oblique X-rays of the knee required for the diagnosis.

Essentially all supracondylar femur fractures require operative intervention because of the severe potential risks of prolonged bedrest.[9] Conservatively management is indicated in cases of nondisplaced or incomplete fractures, impacted stable fracture in elderly, unstable not amenable to fixation due to poor bone quality or gross communication or where surgery is contraindicated. Closed reduction is maintained by continuous traction with the knee in slight flexion and becomes firm rapidly as the fracture is in the cancellous bone. Managed by skin traction on Thomas splint for 6–12 weeks followed by hinged knee brace. Protected weight-bearing with the hinged brace can be initiated.

Active ankle foot exercises starts immediately and knee movements after a few days to avoid redisplacement. It should be gentle and slow.

After 4/6 weeks functional cast bracing and partial weight-bearing is allowed until consolidation, i.e. can bear full weight in the cast brace without any discomfort for 10 second. Full weight-bearing is allowed after 12 weeks in cast brace and brace is discarded after consolidation, 6 months.

Complications of nonoperative management are angular deformity, stiffness, joint incongruity, delayed patient mobility.

Operative management is indicated in cases of displacement. Surgical fixation can be achieved by 95° fixed angle blade plate, dynamic condylar screw, condylar buttress plates, intramedullary nail or rush nails through each femoral condyle, etc. Dynamic condylar screw is less technically demanding than blade plate, blade plate offers most rigid fixation. Antegrade or retrograde intramedullary nailing is selected if the distal fragment is large enough to place a distal interlocking screw. Open fractures require external fixation. Less invasive stabilization system (LISS) provides adequate stable fixation and facilitates healing in mechanically unstable, high-energy fractures of the distal femur.[10]

Postoperatively, active and passive movements start immediately and immediate protected partial weight-bearing is allowed. If rigidity of fixation is doubtful, skin traction is applied for a few weeks post-operatively.

Complications

1. Damage to quadriceps, skin, popliteal artery, etc.
2. Knee stiffness, full range of motion is rarely achieved
3. Nonunion (septic nonunion and aseptic nonunion)
4. Malunion
5. Infection
6. Secondary post-traumatic osteoarthritis.

FRACTURE FEMORAL CONDYLES

Direct injury or fall from a height may drive the tibia up into the intercondylar fossa of femur. One condyle may be fractured and driven upwards or both condyles split apart by the "T" or "Y"-shaped fracture line. Fracture line extends into the joint, so there develops hemarthrosis and severe pain.

Reduction is possible by traction and manual compression, and then the limb is supported in a Thomas splint in continuous skin traction or full length plaster. Managing conservatively good function is regained.

Unicondylar fracture is also possible in femur. Lateral condyle is involved three times as often as the medial one. The physiological valgus causes an abduction component, which explains the greater frequency of lateral condyle fracture.[11] Medial condyle fracture and displacement upwards results in genu varum and lateral condyle in genu valgum. As fracture involves the articular surface, early secondary osteoarthritis may develop.

If reduction not possible by closed means or prolonged immobilization is contradicted, ORIF is indicated. One condyle is fixed by cancellous screw fixation and both the condyles are fixed by right angle nail plate fixation.

Following ORIF immobilization is given by skin traction in Thomas splint for 3–6 weeks followed by nonweight-bearing knee exercises and gait by crutches. Protected partial weight-bearing with the fracture brace can be initiated after 3 months.

Coronal fractures of the femoral condyle (Hoffa fractures) are uncommon injuries that have a better outcome when treated surgically. Postoperatively, all patients began unrestricted immediate ROM. Initial weight-bearing status was limited, but all patients were allowed full weight-bearing within 10 weeks.[12]

FRACTURE TIBIAL CONDYLES

Fracture tibial condyle is more common in elderly. Fractures of the tibial condyles are caused by a combination of vertical thrust and bending (Kennedy and Bailey, 1968). Fracture lateral tibial condyle is more common than medial. It is caused by blow on the side of the knee, i.e. valgus stress. It may be associated with injury to medial collateral ligament, medial meniscus and anterior cruciate ligament. Similar injury on the medial side is not possible to fracture the medial tibial condyle. Fall from a height may also result in fracture one or both the condyles. Occasionally, it is associated with subluxation of whole tibia. Since it is a intra-articular fracture, there develops hemarthrosis and extensive bruising at the site of injury, i.e. on the lateral aspect of knee.

The fate of the joint depends on restoration of satisfactory joint surface, maintenance of the reduction of deformity until bony union and prevention of muscle wasting.

Types of Fracture

Cleavage Condylar Fracture

Oblique fracture line involves the knee joint surface in the inter-condylar area, but weight-bearing articular cartilage is not involved. Compression of the cancellous bone and angular deformity occurs. Vertical fracture line commences across the articular surface of the condyle. Fracture segment gets separated and there is no depression. Tried with closed manipulation and plaster immobilization. No weight-bearing is allowed till union over. Open reduction and internal fixation by screw may be considered.

Depressed Condylar Fracture

Femoral condyle has been driven into the middle of the articular surface of tibial condyle, which is comminuted and depressed, cancellous bone deep to it severely compressed. The remainder of the condyle lateral to it is split off giving rise to widening of tibial plateau.

It is not possible to restore the normal joint surface by conservative means, however good function is achieved.

Plaster immobilization is given following manipulation under anesthesia to correct angular deformity and improve joint surface. No weight-bearing is allowed before 6 weeks. Plaster is removed after 10–12 weeks followed by physiotherapy to improve joint mobility, muscle strength and functions.

Alternatively skin traction though tibia about 15 cm below the joint line can be given for 4–6 weeks to reduce and immobilize the fracture. Immediately passive/active assisted knee movements can be started. Traction corrects displacement and early movements smoothen the articular surface followed by nonweight-bearing exercises and gait training.

Open reduction—depressed fragment is elevated and the underlying gap is filled with bone graft from ileum. Overcorrected fracture fragment is fixed with screw followed by early nonweight-bearing movements.

Comminuted Fracture

Comminuted fracture can be managed by skin traction and early movements or open reduction and internal fixation.

FRACTURE BOTH BONES OF LEG

Fracture both bones of leg is usually caused by twisting force or direct blow. Rotational/twisting force results in spiral fracture at different levels, tibia at middle and lower 3rd junction and fibula at middle and upper 3rd junction. Angulatory force from direct blow results in transverse or short oblique fracture at the same level.

1. As a rule there is considerable displacement and redisplacement
2. High incidence of open and infected fracture because tibia lies superficially beneath the skin
3. Cosmetic and functional disability because of malalignment, foot faced externally
4. Slow union because of poor vascularity.

Isolated fracture shaft of fibula occurs from direct violence causing little functional incapacity as it serves only for attachment of muscles and bears no weight.

So, only immobilization is given till pain subsides and then walking is allowed with crepe bandage. Sometimes BK walking plaster is given for 3–4 weeks.

Fracture of upper shaft or neck of fibula is associated with rupture of medial collateral ligament, whereas fracture lower shaft is associated with dislocation of ankle.

Closed fracture tibia can be managed by closed reduction and long plaster cast immobilization for 12 weeks. Unreduced fracture or open fracture requires initial calcaneal traction for 2 weeks so that wound heals, swelling subsides. Then ORIF can be done, it takes 24 weeks for consolidation.

Immediately ankle foot toes and knee movements should be encouraged. Functional cast bracing may be given after 6-8 weeks. Then partial weight-bearing is allowed.

Undisplaced stable fracture tibia (transverse or long oblique) can be managed by immobilization in long leg cast with rocker bottom. Walking is allowed after 2/3 weeks once the initial reaction is over. Long leg cast is replaced by balloon kyphoplasty (BK) walking plaster after 4/6 weeks.

Displaced fracture is reduced under anesthesia. If stable after reduction, is managed by long leg plaster cast immobilization with rocker bottom, which is replaced by BK walking cast after 8 weeks. Walking is allowed after 4/6 weeks.

Displaced unstable fracture/comminuted fracture can be managed by skin traction though calcaneus for a few weeks followed by long leg plaster with the traction for 8/12 weeks or only traction for 10–12 weeks.

During immobilization, static quadriceps and gastrosoleus contraction, SLR for hip abduction, adduction, flexion and extension freely and then resisted should be done to prevent atrophy.

Foot support should be provided to prevent tightness of TA. Toes pressing against the support, toes parting and closing, static PF exercise, foot shortening and lengthening for lumbrical exercise, etc. help in prevention of flat foot and equines foot.

Walks with limping, may be habitual/acquired while the limb was in plaster, pain at the site/sole of foot, weakness of muscles, stiffness of ankle foot and knee, fear, coordination defect due to general weakness, etc. Pain at the site, sole of foot arises from the short plantar fascia and ligaments, atrophy of intrinsics, clawing of toes, adhesion, etc.

Plaster cast during immobilization supports the vessel wall, following plaster removal due to lack of support to the vessel wall by the skeletal muscle tone, dense fibrous deep fascia and vasomotor tone gives rise to edema lower limb. Loss of external as well as internal support to the vessel wall results in vasodilatation and edema. It requires vigorous strengthening exercises to build-up the muscle tone and support to the vessel wall to check vasodilatation and edema.

Following plaster removal, mobility, strengthening, stretching, coordination exercises followed by functional re-education are given.

Indication for ORIF is grossly unstable and reducible fracture. Screw fixation or wiring is done for oblique or spiral fracture. Full weight-bearing plaster cast is applied after 2/3 weeks and maintained for 10–12 weeks. Plate and screw fixation, if rigid, 2/3 weeks bed rest and nonweight-bearing exercises are advised, then long leg walking plaster cast and nonweight-bearing crutch walking is allowed.

IMN is rigid fixation, so nonweight-bearing knee movements can be initiated after 2 weeks, partial weight-bearing after 8 weeks and full weight-bearing after 12 weeks.

External fixator is indicated for comminuted fracture, open injury. Nonweight-bearing can be started after 2 weeks.

Complications

1. Vascular complication is characterized by pain on distal and medial side of calf. Pain on passive toes extension, active flexion of toes and plantar hyposthesia.
2. Compartment syndrome
3. Popliteal artery could be stretched by proximal fracture segment in case of fracture proximal third of tibia.
4. Neurological complication could be stretching of posterior tibial nerve.
5. Nonunion/delayed union and malunion.

DISLOCATION OF KNEE

Historically knee dislocation has been a rare event. Kennedy found only two knee dislocations among 700,000 injuries reported to the workman's compensation board of Ontario, for the year 1955 to 1957. A survey of 140,231 admissions to two large Philadelphia hospitals revealed only two cases of knee dislocation. Only 14 cases of knee dislocation were found in a review of more than 2 million admissions to the Mayo Clinic, from 1911 to 1960.

The classification of knee dislocation is based primarily on the position of the displaced tibia on the femur. The four main categories are anterior, posterior, medial and lateral. In the case where the knee presents in a reduced position, the dislocation is classified according to the direction of the instability. Rotational instability represents the fifth category, which is further classified into anteromedial, anterolateral, posteromedial and posterolateral.

Current classification of dislocation of the knee based on the extent of ligamentous injury.[13]

Classification Associated Ligamentous Injury

KD-I :	Dislocation without both cruciate involved
KD-II:	Dislocation with bicruciate disruption only
KD-III:	Dislocation with bicruciate + posteromedial or postero-lateral disruption
KD-IV:	Dislocation with bicruciate + posteromedial and postero-lateral disruption
KD-V:	Dislocation with fracture
KD-V1:	Dislocation without both cruciates involved
KD-V2:	Bicruciate disruption only
KD-V3M:	Bicruciate + posteromedial disruption
KD-V3L:	Bicruciate + posterolateral disruption
KD-V4:	Posteromedial and posterolateral disruption.

The anterior dislocation is the most common type of knee dislocations. 40% of 245 knee dislocations reviewed by Green were anterior, 33% posterior, 18% lateral, 4% medial and 5% rotational. Forced hyperextension is the primary mechanism of injury causing anterior dislocation of the knee. Kennedy found in cadaver knee specimens that at approximately 30° of hyperextension the posterior capsule was first structure to tear, followed by ACL and PCL. At about 50° of hyperextension popliteal artery was found to rupture.

The most common mechanism of posterior dislocation is the motor vehicle accident. During abrupt deceleration the dash board strikes the anterior tibia while the knee is flexed. This translates the tibia posteriorly on the femur. Considerably more force is required to dislocate the knee by this mechanism compared with the hyperextension mechanism for anterior dislocation. 75–100 inch-pound placed on anterior tibia of a cadaver knee has been found to be the force necessary to rupture the PCL alone and up to 800 inch-pound is necessary to dislocate the knee posteriorly. ACL is also injured, but there is evidence of intact ACL in case of posterior dislocation. 44% of posterior dislocation have been found to have injury to the popliteal artery. The posteriorly directed tibia directly compresses the popliteal artery and can transect it.

The mechanism of injury in medial and lateral knee dislocations are primarily the result of a forceful blow to medial or lateral side of the knee while the foot is fixed on the ground. The blow creates extreme varus or valgus moment on the knee. Disruption of the collateral ligaments and cruciate ligament is seen medial or lateral dislocation resulting in multidirectional instability. Injury to the peroneal nerve is commonly seen in lateral dislocation, owing to the anatomical vulnerability as it runs lateral to the fibular head. Injury to the nerve ranges from neuropraxia to complete transaction. Complete rupture of the nerve was most commonly found in dislocations with combined complete disruption of the ACL, PCL and posterolateral corner.

Neurological injury: Palsy of the common peroneal nerve was associated with dislocation of the knee in 25% of our series of 55 patients, exclusively with dislocations involving a disruption of the PCL and posterolateral corner. Tibial plateau and supracondylar femur fractures may be associated.

Vascular injury: The popliteal artery is tethered proximally by the adductor hiatus of the thigh and distally by the fascial arch of proximal soleus. It is susceptible to injury during knee dislocation, either by direct blow or by stretch. The incidence of vascular injury in knee dislocation ranges up to 40%. Knee dislocation patients with signs or symptoms of vascular injury but without limb threatening ischemia may require arteriography. Spasm, thrombosis, or propagation of an intimal tear of the popliteal artery may lead to vascular compromise. Monitoring must be consistent and pulses must be checked hourly. Obvious vascular compromise and limb threatening ischemia after knee dislocation should be treated with immediate vascular repair of the popliteal artery.[14]

Neurological injuries: The incidence of vascular injury in knee dislocation ranges up to 40%.

Evaluation

History of mechanism of injury and position of the injured limb at the time of accident may provide clues to the possible ligamentous involvement. Integrity of the skin is assessed and any open injuries found that complicate the type and timing of subsequent treatment. Detail neurovascular evaluations are documented. Special tests to check the integrity of ACL, PCL, collateral ligaments must be done. After initial clinical evaluation plane radiographs, magnetic resonance imaging, computerized tomography and complex motion tomography are done for the evaluation of surrounding soft tissues and osseous structures. Arteriography for the diagnosis of vascular injury and electromyographic studies for the diagnosis of nerve injury should be performed.

Management

The initial treatment of knee dislocations in the 20th century focused on cast immobilization. Mitchell in 1930 recommended 4-6 weeks immobilization to allow complete soft tissue healing. In 1937 Conwell and Alldredge and later Griswold, in 1951, immobilized the knee for 6-10 weeks but started quadriceps muscle sets immediately to avoid muscle atrophy.

In 1967 Myles found in a series of 7 knee dislocations that the final range of motion was inversely proportional to the length of immobilization. He recommended only 2 weeks of cast immobilization in uncompleted knee dislocation in which reduction was routine. In 1972, Taylor et al. studied 42 knee dislocations in which 26 were treated nonoperatively with cast immobilization from 3 to 12 weeks. 16 knees underwent open reduction, 3 of these had primary repair of injured ligaments. 40 of the patients received follow-up from 6 months to 35 years later. Conservative treatment yielded 18 of 26 good results. Operative treatment yielded 4 of 16 good results. Conservative treatment was recommended as the method of choice with immobilization no longer than 6 weeks. In a 1996 review of literature, Henshaw et al. states that knee dislocation has been a matter of controversy with regard to the need for ligamentous reconstruction.

Repair of ligamentous injuries after closed reduction was first described in the 1950s and became an acceptable, alternative method of treatment of knee dislocations in the 1960s and 70s. In 1955, O'Donoghue described the results of operative repair of 80 mixed knee ligamentous injuries. Direct repair by suturing of the ligaments end to end for midsubstance tears and end to bone with avulsions led to consistently good result. Consistently better results were realized when operative repair was performed within 2 weeks of the initial injury.

In 1963, Kennedy reviewed 22 cases of knee dislocation. 6 of the patients underwent repair of injured ligamentous structures acutely from 2 hours to 1 week after injury and found that repair of ligamentous structures had resulted in useful knees. In 1969, Shields et al. studied 26 knee dislocations in which operative repair of injured ligamentous structures was performed in 12 cases and nonoperative treatment was administered in 14 cases. Operative treatment led to better results than nonoperative treatment at a follow up range of 3 months to 27 years.

In 1971, Meyers and Harvey studied 18 knee dislocations. Operative repair of injured ligamentous structures was performed in 11 of 18 cases. The knees with ligamentous injury that were treated nonoperatively had developed instability on follow up. Immediate closed reduction and early operative repair of all damaged ligaments were recommended. If vascular repair was undertaken, repair of ligaments was delayed 3–4 weeks. Postoperative cast immobilization was used for 6 weeks, followed by 6 weeks of protected weight-bearing. Four years later Meyers and colleagues found 13 of 16 good results with repair of all injured ligaments and 1 of 13 good results with cast immobilization. They concluded that operative repair of all injured ligamentous structures led to the best results.

In 1971, Jones et al. studied 22 patients with knee dislocations. Operative repair was performed in 14 of 22 ligament injuries and 8 of 22 were treated nonoperatively. At a follow up to 2-12 months after injury showed repair of torn ligaments offers the best chance of a stable knee.

In 1985, Sisto and warren studied 22 patients with knee dislocations, in which acute operative repair of all torn ligaments was performed on 13 knees. Semitendinosis or gracilis graft reinforcements were used in midsubstance cruciate tears. Cast immobilization was used for 4 weeks after cast immobilization was used for 6 weeks care. 77% of operative patients returned to sporting activities. They recommended acute repair of ligamentous injury in young active patients to allow earlier motion and return to activities. Manipulation under anesthesia to gain range of motion was recommended if the patient had less than 90° range of motion at 12 weeks.

In 1984, Thomson et al. performed early operative repair of torn ligaments in 6 of 10 patients and cast immobilization in 4 of 10 patients. All knees were immobilized for 6 weeks in plaster. At 6 years follow up, good results were obtained in 3 of 5 operated cases and in 2 of 5 nonoperated cases. They concluded that operative and conservative treatment led to similar results. Operative treatment was recommended only in cases with pronounced instability.

In 1987, Montgomery reviewed the literature on ligament injury and repair in knee dislocation. He concluded that surgical and nonsurgical approaches would yield good results but added that excellent or near excellent results are unlikely to be obtained unless operative repair is undertaken. He, therefore, recommended early repair of ligament injury in young active patients, 10–12 days after arterial repair. Postoperatively, a hinged knee brace was recommended at 40°–70° for first 8 weeks and then 10°–90° for 4 more weeks.

In 1987, Roman and colleagues reviewed 30 patients with knee dislocations with follow up on 20 patients. They found the operative knees to have greater stability but with greater loss of range of motion. This result was attributed to prolonged immobilization (>6 weeks) with transarticular pin fixation.

In 1991, Frassica et al. treated 17 patients with knee dislocations. 13 patients underwent early surgery within 5 days of injury. Both operative and nonoperative groups were cast immobilized of externally fixated for a mean of 55 days. All the 12 patients were noted to have good or excellent results.

In 1991, Shelbourne and colleagues reported on operative intervention for 20 low energy sports related knee dislocation with early reconstruction of the PCL with autologous bone-patella-bone graft. 77% of patients returned to sporting activities, but only 19% returned to premorbid level of competition. They also found that when ACL reconstruction was delayed longer than 3 weeks, patients had a much lower incidence of arthrofibrosis and an earlier return of strength. In 1994, Walker et al. treated 13 knee dislocations in the same way as Shelbourne and recommended early reconstruction of the PCL and late reconstruction of the ACL if instability persisted.

In 1999, Yeh et al. reported 22 of 23 knee dislocations who underwent early arthroscopic reconstruction of the PCL with autologous bone-patella-bone graft and debridement of ACL. The surgery were undertaken once the inflammation subsided, mean 11.1 days after injury. All the patients were protected by knee brace for 3 weeks followed by progressive range of motion up to 3 months. At follow up after a mean of 27 months, all the patients showed have good results.

In 1995, Shapiro and Freedman retrospectively reviewed 7 openly reconstructed combined ACL-PCL injuries. The reconstructions were performed by allograft patella tendon or Achilles' tendon at an average of 9.6 days after injury. All the patients were placed in knee brace allowing 0-70 of motion. Early ROM exercise by CPM machine and protected weight bearing were begun immediately after surgery. 4 patients developed arthrofibrosis and manipulation at a mean of 17 weeks after surgery. The result showed 3 of 7 excellent, 3 good and 1 fair result.

In 1996, Fanelli et al. presented 20 arthroscopically assisted ACL-PCL reconstructions with either allograft Achilles' tendon or autograft patella tendon. The result showed significant improvement. In 1997, Noyes and Barber-Westin described arthroscopic reconstructions of combined ACL-PCL injuries in 11 patients. The result at follow up after mean of 4.8 years showed 1 of 7 excellent, 2 good, 1 fair and 3 poor results.

In 1999, Wascher et al. retrospectively reviewed 13 patients with knee dislocations, who underwent early, open reconstruction of ACL-PCL with allograft. Nonweight-bearing with hinged knee brace (20-70) was maintained for 6 weeks followed by full weight-bearing and full range of motion. At a mean of 38 months, average range of motion was 130 with minor extension and flexion losses. 6 patients returned to unrestricted sports activities and 4 patients returned to modified sports.

In a recent large study of injury to the peroneal nerve from a variety of causes, the results of nerve grafting were poor when grafts in excess of 6 cm were required.[14]

Dislocation of the knee results in severe soft-tissue disruption and although modern surgical techniques and better understanding of these injuries have improved the outcome, a return to normal function is uncommon.

Although the range of movement and functional outcome scores are better in patients treated by ligamentous reconstruction rather than nonsurgical treatment, some residual impairment of function is expected. The most common complications after surgical repair are joint stiffness and failure of some component of the reconstruction. In one long-term evaluation of outcome, dislocation was associated with a risk of post-traumatic osteoarthritis of 50%.[13]

Congenital Dislocation of Knee

The incidence of congenital dislocation of knee is estimated to be 1 in 100,00 live births. This is 80 times rarer than congenital dislocation of hip. Women are more affected than men, and blacks have a rarer incidence than whites. Congenital talipes equinovarus (CTEV) and bilateral congenital hip dislocation (CDH) are commonly found in association with congenital dislocation of knee.

Congenital dislocation of knee is a hyperextension deformity of the knee that presents at birth. It is believed to be the result of a genetic abnormality or poor intrauterine positioning. A breech position and oligohydramnios have been cited as causes of this condition.

The altered anatomy of the knee includes fibrosis of the quadriceps, an ablated suprapatellar pouch, anterior cruciate elongation, dysplasia of the articular surfaces and displacement of hamstrings anteriorly.

Treatment includes serial casting biweekly until reduction is achieved. If progress is not made with serial casting, operative management is indicated. Surgery consists of quadriceps lengthening, capsular releases and posterior transfer of hamstring tendons to achieve reduction.

REFERENCES

1. Chelsea H. Neuromuscular electrical stimulation and quadriceps strength following patellar fracture and open reduction internal fixation surgery: a case report. 2015. Case Report Papers. Paper 34.
2. IbounigT, Simons TA. Etiology, diagnosis and treatment of tendinous knee extensor mechanism Injuries. Scand J Surg. 2016;105(2):67-72.
3. Negrin LL, Nemecek E, Hajdu S. Extensor mechanism ruptures of the knee: differences in demographic data and long-term outcome after surgical treatment. Injury. 2015;46(10):1957-63.
4. Petri M, Liodakis E, Hofmeister M, Despang FJ, Maier M, Balcarek P, et al. Operative vs conservative treatment of traumatic patellar dislocation: results of a prospective randomized controlled clinical trial. Arch Orthop Trauma Surg. 2013;133(2): 209-13.
5. Roth S, Madarevic T, Vukelic L, Roth A, Madarevic DG, Cicvaric T. Influence of arthroscopic lateral release on functional recovery in adolescents with recurrent patellar dislocation. Archiv Orthop Trauma Surg. 2013;133(10):1441-5.
6. Petri M, et al. current concept for patellar dislocation. Arch Trauma Res. 2015;4(3):e29301.

7. Fulkerson JP. Surgical correction of recurrent patella instability. Healio Orthopedics Today. 2007.

8. Paterno MV, et al. Early rehabilitation following surgical fixation of a femoral shaft fracture. Phys Ther. 2006;86(4):558-72.

9. Rabin SI. Supracondylar femur fractures treatment & management. 2015.

10. Weight M, Collinge C. Early results of the less invasive stabilization system for mechanically unstable fractures of the distal femur (AO/OTA Types A2, A3, C2, and C3). J Orthop Trauma. 2004;18(8):503-8.

11. Holmes SM, Bomback D, Baumgaertner MR. Coronal fractures of the femoral condyle: a brief report of five cases. J Orthop Trauma. 2004;18(5):316-9.

12. Manfredini M, Gildone A, Ferrante R, Bernasconi S, Massari L. Unicondylar femoral fractures: therapeutic strategy and long-term results. A Review of 23 Patients. 2001;67(2):132-8.

13. Robertson A, Nutton RW, Keating JF. Dislocation of the knee. J Bone Joint Surg Br. 2006;88(6);706-11.

14. Niall DM, Nutton RW, Keating JF. Palsy of the common peroneal nerve after traumatic dislocation of the knee. J Bone Joint Surg. 2005; 87(5):664-7.

Chapter 6

Physiotherapy in Surgical Conditions

SYNOVECTOMY

Surgical excision of the synovial membrane lining the joint is known as synovectomy. The surgical procedure can be performed arthroscopically or by opening the joint to remove the synovial tissue surrounding the joint that has become inflamed and swollen.[1]

Indications

1. Rheumatoid arthritis and osteoarthritis, not responding to conservative management
2. Pigmented villonodular synovitis (PVNS)[2]
3. Synovial hypertrophy and joint pain secondary to recurrent hemarthrosis as the result of hemophilia[3]
4. Synovial osteochondromatosis[4]
5. Infectious synovitis as in tuberculosis
6. Severe pain
7. Before damage to articular surface.

Type

1. *Open synovectomy:* The surgery is performed through antero-medial incision. Opening up the rear of the knee to remove the synovial lining in the back of the joint was sometimes done as a more radical extension of the frontal synovectomy procedure. These open surgical procedures had serious drawbacks, in that they were quite painful and often produced major postoperative morbidity such as joint scarring and stiffness.[5]
2. *Arthroscopic synovectomy:* Arthroscopic synovectomy involves the use of multiple portals for access to and endoscopic removal of as much synovium as possible from all compartments of the knee.[6]

3. *Radiosynovectomy:* Radiosynovectomy is a novel method of treatment for several acute and chronic inflammatory joint disorders. A small amount of a beta-emitting radionuclide is injected into the affected joint delivering a radiation dose of 70 to 100 Gy to the synovia. The proliferative tissue is destroyed, secretion of fluid and accumulation of inflammation causing cellular compounds stops and the joint surfaces become fibrosed, providing long-term symptom relief.[7]

4. *Chemical synovectomy:* Chemical synovectomy utilizing intra-articular injection of osmium tetroxide (osmic acid) or alkylation agents has been used to perform a "medical synovectomy" in patients with synovial inflammation due to various disorders, including rheumatoid arthritis, psoriatic arthritis, pigmented villonodular synovitis, and ankylosing spondylitis.[8]

Arthroscopic synovectomy was just as good and probably better than open surgical synovectomy in chronic inflammatory synovitis of the knee.[9]

Procedure

Postoperative Physiotherapy following Surgical Synovectomy

Knee immobilized by compressive dressing to prevent/manage postsurgical joint effusion.

❑ Immediate postoperatively active ankle foot and toes movements, static quadriceps exercise and straight leg raise (SLR) are encouraged

❑ Partial weight bearing walking with brace and crutches can be started from 1st day

❑ Active knee movements are initiated after 48–72 hours

❑ Knee mobilization and progressive strengthening can start after stitch removal so that full range and adequate strength can be achieved by 6th weeks and then patient returns to activities.

Postoperative Physiotherapy following Arthroscopic Synovectomy

❑ Immediately, knee immobilized by compressive dressing and in elevation, apply ice 20 minutes 5–6 times for day for 48-72 hours, active ankle foot and toes movements, static quadriceps exercise and SLR. Electrical stimulation to quadriceps can be given.

Active range of motion (ROM) exercise can be initiated on first day, so that full knee extension and 90° of flexion can be achieved by 10–12 days.

❑ Protected weightbearing with the knee brace and crutches is allowed by 5–7 days.

Return to work: If patients' job involves sitting for the majority of the day they can return after 3 days. If their job is physically demanding and involve heavy manual work or standing for long periods then 1-2 weeks off work may be necessary.[10,11]

KNEE REPLACEMENT (FIG. 6.1)

Total knee replacement (TKR) or total knee arthroplasty (TKA), is a surgical procedure in which parts of the knee joint are replaced with artificial parts (prostheses).

A normal knee functions as a hinge joint between the upper leg bone (femur) and the lower leg bones (tibia and fibula). The surfaces where these bones meet can become worn out overtime, often due to arthritis or other conditions, which can cause pain and swelling.[12]

As of 2010, over 600,000 total knee replacements were being performed annually in the United States and were increasingly common. Among older patients in the US, the per capita number of primary total knee replacements doubled from 1991 to 2010 (from 31 to 62 per 10,000 Medicare enrollees annually). The number of total knee replacements performed annually in the US is expected to grow by 6.73% to 3.48 million procedures by 2030.

Women are more likely to undergo TKAs than men with a ratio of 1.4/1, which was the same ratio 15 years ago.[13]

The main indication for TKA is OA, which accounts for more than 94 to 97% of TKA operations.[14,15]

Recent advances have increased the success of knee replacement surgery. Researches in the areas of biomechanical alignment, fixation methods, material implementation, postoperative management has led to improvement in function. Postoperative physiotherapy is important to reduce the morbidity of surgery. So therapist should know the component employed and their surgical implementation, etc.

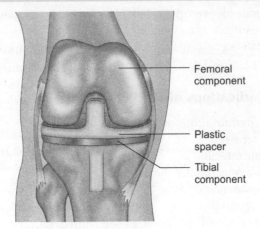

Fig. 6.1: Total knee replacement

(*Source:* Revision Total Knee Replacement. http://orthoinfo.aaos.org/topic. cfm?topic=A00712).

Indications of TKR[16,17]

❑ Osteoarthritis of knee[18,23]
❑ Rheumatoid arthritis
❑ Job traumatic arthritis
❑ Osteochondromatosis
❑ Villonodular synovitis
❑ Metabolic arthritis
❑ Osteonecrosis
❑ Gout, pseudogout
❑ Walking, going up stairs and getting in and out of chairs is difficult
❑ Pain is moderate to severe even while resting and may affect sleep
❑ Joint degeneration has caused knee deformity, such as bow-legs or knock-knees.
❑ Swelling and inflammation is chronic and not controlled with medication or rest.

In December 2003, the National Institutes of Health (NIH) in the United States published a consensus statement on TKR (based on the Agency Healthcare Research and Quality's Technology Assessment), concluded that the indications for TKR should include these:

❑ Radiologic evidence of joint damage

❑ Moderate to severe persistent pain that is not adequately relieved by nonsurgical management
❑ Clinically significant functional limitation resulting in diminished quality.

Contraindications of TKR[19,24]

Absolute contraindications include:
❑ Knee sepsis
❑ Chronic infection
❑ Extensor mechanism dysfunction
❑ Severe vascular disease
❑ Recurvatum deformity secondary to muscular weakness
❑ Presence of well-functioning knee arthrodesis.

Relative and controversial contraindications include:
❑ Medical conditions that preclude safe anesthesia
❑ Inadequate soft tissue coverage
❑ Morbid obesity
❑ Neuropathic arthropathy
❑ History of osteomyelitis around knee joint.

Procedure of TKR

Partial

McIntosh: Part or both the tibial condyles are removed and replaced by metal disc, to which femur articulates.

Sledge

Replacement of either medial/lateral compartment of tibiofemoral articulation is achieved by inserting a metal runner on the appropriate femoral condyle, which glides with polyethylene component of adjacent tibial condyle.

The components are secured by bone cement. Outcome of it is less satisfactory and more uncertain than that of hip replacement arthroplasty because it is a superficial joint, so there is more chance of infection. It is a complex joint biomechanically, i.e. it is a polycentric joint and there is gliding as well as rolling occur during knee flexion-extension. Unless design of the prosthesis permits gliding and rotational movements as well as hinging, torsional force will be produced and loosen the prosthesis.

Types of Prosthesis

The type of prosthesis offered depends upon the patient's age, weight, gender, anatomy, activity level, medical history, and general health.[21, 25]

Constrained Joint (also called hinged)

❏ This is the most common type of knee replacement prosthesis
❏ Simple hinge, in which the femoral and tibial components are stemmed and also linked together to allow only hinging movements
❏ This prosthesis is used when a patient's ligaments and muscles are not able to provide stability for the knee prosthesis.

Advantage: Prosthesis itself is stable, does not depend on knee ligament for stability.

Disadvantage: It is exposed to torsional force resulting in loosening of prosthesis.
❏ Require excision of large amount of bone for the insertion of prosthesis, which makes arthrodesis difficult as salvage procedure.

Unconstrained Joint

Surfaces of the tibia and femur are covered by polyethylene and metal respectively with no linkage of the components.

Advantages: Rotation and gliding minimize torsion, so no chance of loosening of prosthesis.
❏ Lesser bone excision is required for the insertion of prosthesis so if the replacement fails hinged prosthesis or arthrodesis can be performed as a salvage procedure. It depends on the ligament for stability.

Semiconstrained Joint

The prosthesis comprise of two components with a linkage system, which is not rigid like a simple hinge, so it is stable and at the same time it permits some freedom of rotation and gliding movements to minimize the torsion.

Incision: Anterior midline/medial parapateller incision.

Anterior midline (midvastus) approach is considered as muscle sparing technique with a deep dissection exposing VMO. Medial parapatellar incision is most commonly used approach which stretches and compromises the integrity of extensor mechanism.

There are 3 options for holding the knee replacement prosthesis in place:

1. *Cemented fixation procedure:* It fixes the prosthesis to the bones with polymethyl methacrylate. The cement allows the prosthesis to fit perfectly to the bone, even if there are bone irregularities. A cemented knee replacement stabilizes rapidly, so patients can walk (i.e. bear weight on the joint) immediately following surgery. The disadvantage is that if the cement loosens, then bone may be ground away by movement of the joint, making subsequent revisions difficult.

2. *Non-cemented procedure:* Uses a prosthesis with a rough porous surface that is designed to let bone grow into it, thus eliminating the need for cement. The prosthesis is fitted precisely next to the bone and fixed into place with metal pegs and screws while the bone grows and fixes to the knee replacement prosthesis. As would be expected, there is a longer recovery time to walking (i.e. weight-bearing) compared to using cemented prostheses.

   The advantage is that if the prosthesis does loosen overtime, then less bone loss occurs due to the lack of the irritant cement.

3. *Hybrid fixation:* It is a combination of cemented and noncemented procedures. The femur is cemented, while the tibia is not. Hybrid fixation and noncemented procedures are relatively new procedures, and the long-term outcomes of patients undergoing these types of fixation technique are unknown. At this time, most knee replacement surgeries use the cemented procedure.

   The Ontario Joint Replacement Registry (OJRR) annual report from 2004 reported that 80% of the knee replacements were cemented, 13% were hybrids, and 7% were non-cemented.[26]

Physical Assessment

Age, medical conditions (pain, effusion) pre-exiting severity of arthritis, type of gait and walking aid, surrounding soft tissue instability, tightness/contracture, muscle strength, patient's social habits, occupational needs, degree of axial alignment to be corrected, type of prosthesis to be employed, fixation method, goal of the patient, etc. should be evaluated. Patient must be explained about the surgery, expected postoperative outcome, potential risk and complication, etc. Pre and postoperative physiotherapy regimen should be carried out.

Postoperatively patient's overall medical conditions such as cardiopulmonary and circulatory must be evaluated. The aim is to prevent/minimize/correct postoperative complications, restoration of motion and strength, and early return to activity.

Radiographic Assessment[22,27]

An appropriate musculoskeletal radiologic study is essential in planning of TKR. The presence of bone defects might be detected and preoperative decision whether to use a primary or revision implant should be given. Determination of the joint line is also important in determining the flexion/extension space and balance of the ligaments. Tracking of the quadriceps mechanism and rotational deformities are other important issues for patellar stability, however may not be assessed on direct radiographs especially in deformed knees with fixed valgus position. Conventional radiographs are usually adequate for initial radiographic evaluation to confirm the diagnosis or assess the severity of the disease. Preoperative radiographic planning for total knee arthroplasty begins by obtaining a high quality standing anteroposterior (AP) and lateral 52-inch cassette graphics. Additional views such as Merchant, tunnel, patella sunrise, orthoroentgenogram or advanced imaging modalities such as CT, MRI may be necessary in extraordinary conditions such as congenital dislocation of the patella, post-traumatic deformities, severe deformities, tumors and congenital anomalies.

Risks and Complications in Knee Replacement

Deep vein thrombosis (DVT): According to the American Academy of Orthopedic Surgeons (AAOS), deep vein thrombosis in the leg is the most common complication of knee replacement surgery... prevention... may include periodic elevation of patient's legs, lower leg exercises to increase circulation, support stockings and medication to thin your blood.[28]

Persistent pain or stiffness: Occurs in 8–23% of patients. Prosthesis failure occurs in approximately 2% of patients at 5 years.[29]

Fracture: Periprosthetic fractures are becoming more frequent with the aging patient population and can occur intraoperatively or postoperatively.

Nerve injuries: Occur in 1–2% of patients. Persistent pain or stiffness occurs in 8–23% of patients.[30]

Loss of motion: The knee at times may not recover its normal range of motion (0–135° usually) after total knee replacement.

Infection: The current classification of AAOS divides prosthetic infections into four types:[31]

1. *Type 1 (positive intraoperative culture):* Positive intraoperative cultures.
2. *Type 2 (early postoperative infection):* Infection occurring within first month after surgery
3. *Type 3 (acute hematogenous infection):* Hematogenous seeding of site of previously well-functioning prosthesis.
4. *Type 4 (late chronic infection):* Chronic indolent clinical course; infection present for more than a month.

While it is relatively rare, periprosthetic infection remains one of the most challenging complications of joint arthroplasty.

Obesity: There is increased risk in complications for obese people going through total knee replacement.[32] The morbidly obese should be advised to lose weight before surgery and, if medically eligible, would probably benefit from bariatric surgery.

Postoperative Physiotherapy

Phase I—Early Motion

Early motion helps to reduce joint swelling, pain, restore motion, etc. Patellar mobilization can start after 48 hours.

- Ankle pumping exercises with the leg elevated immediately/after surgery to prevent a DVT or pulmonary embolism
- Deep breathing exercises
- Isometric exercises for quadriceps, hamstrings, hip abductors, adductors and extensors can be started early.

- SLR for hip flexion, abduction, adduction can be given earlier in case of cemented and after 6-8 weeks in case of uncemented prosthesis. Extension can be initiated as prone lying is tolerated
- Range of motion exercise can be given by continuous passive motion (CPM) from 10°-15° to 70°-90°, as pain allows, in the recovery room with the hinge brace adjusted from 0° to 90° position.
- Number of studies describing the benefits of CPM, such as decreased need for postoperative pain medication, decreased incidence of DVT, and increased or more rapid recovery of ROM, were reported in the literature.
- Porous self-retaining prosthesis is fixed by bone graft and screw. It requires 2-3 weeks immobilization for the bony ingrowth into the pores of the prosthesis. This correlates to a fracture healing process.
- Usually cement is used at the bone-prosthesis interface for fixation. It gets fixed immediately, so more rapid advance weight-bearing is allowed. Patient can wean from crutches within 4-6 weeks. Factors limiting fare weight bearing are soft tissue healing and postoperative response.

Phase II—Moderate Protection Phase (after 6 weeks)

- Multi-angle isometric quadriceps exercise 90°, 70°, 50°, 30°, 10° and electrical stimulation can be given
- Pool therapy, ROM exercise, static cycling for endurance, resisted quadriceps exercise from 90° to 30° range, stretching, etc. can be given
- In case of cemented, full weight-bearing is allowed after 6 weeks, provided there is no pain, no swelling, is 0°-90° and adequate strength, proprioception and balance.
- In case of uncemented porous prosthesis, 50-75% partial weight bearing is allowed and patient can wean from crutches by 9th weeks
- Balance training starts once full weight-bearing is allowed.

Phase III—Advance Rehabilitative Phase and Activity Phase (after 12 weeks)

Progressive strengthening, stretching exercises for hamstrings, TA, hip external rotators should be given. Mini squat and get up, step climbing, cycling, swimming and progressive walking can be given to improve the endurance. Gradually, patient returns to functional activity by 16–20 weeks.

REFERENCES

1. Wiedel JD. Arthroscopic synovectomy: state of the art. Haemophilia. 2002;8(3):372-4.
2. Mollon B, Lee A.The effect of surgical synovectomy and radiotheraphy on the rate of recurrence pigmented villonodular synovitis of the knee: an individual patient meta-analysis. Bone Joint J. 2015;97-B:550-7.
3. Rampal V , Odent T, et al. Surgical synovectomy of the knee in young haemophiliacs: long-term results of a monocentric series of 23 patients. J Child Orthop. 2010;4(1):33-7.
4. Singh S, et al. Disseminated synovial chonromatosis of knee treated by open radical synovectomy using combined anterior and posterior approaches. 2014.
5. Seepage A. The knee and shoulder. Centre of New Jersey and Pennsylvains. 2007.
6. Patel D. Arthroscopic synovectomy. In: Jackson DW (Ed). Master Techniques in Orthopedic Surgery: Knee Surgery, 2nd edition. Philadelphia: Lippincott Williams & Wilkins, 2003, pp. 417-25.
7. Das BK, et al. Role of radiosynovectomy in the treatment of rheumatoid arthritis and hemophilic arthropathies. Biomed Imaging Interv J. 2007;3(4):e45.
8. Wright RJ, et al. Synovectomy for inflammatory arthritis of the knee.2007.
9. Chalmers PN, et al. Rheumatoid Synovectomy: Does the Surgical Approach Matter? 2010.
10. Royal national orthopaedic hospital knee arthroscopy Guidelines 2010. Review 2012.
11. James H,et al. The Journal of Arthroscopic and Related Surgery. 2008; 24.
12. Martin GM, et al. Total knee replacement (arthroplasty). 2016.
13. Healthcare Cost and Utilization Project. Agency for Healthcare Research and Quality. http://hcupnet.ahrq.gov (Accessed on December 20, 2012).
14. Cram P, Lu X, Kates SL, et al. Total knee arthroplasty volume, utilization, and outcomes among Medicare beneficiaries, 1991-2010.JAMA. 2012;308:1227-37.
15. Kurtz S, Ong K, Lau E, et al. Projections of primary and revision hip and knee arthroplasty in the United States from 2005 to 2030. J Bone Joint Surg Am. 2007;89:780.
16. Culliford Dj, Maskell J, Beard DJ, Murray DW, Price AJ, Arden NK. Temporal trends in hip and knee replacement in the United Kingdom: 1991 to 2006. J Bone Joint Surg Br. 2010;92(1):130-5.

17. National Joint Registry. National Joint Registry for England and Wales:7th Annual Report, 2010. Hertfordshire, England: National Joint Registry; 2008.
18. Robertsson O, Bizjajeva S, Fenstad AM, et al. Knee arthroplasty in Denmark, Norway and Sweden. Acta Orthop.2010;81(1):82-8.
19. Borzic KJ. Total knee replacement for knee arthritis. 2013.
20. Erdogan AO, Gokay NS, et al. Preoperative planning of total knee replacement. 2013.
21. Mike D, Van Manen, et al. Management of primary knee osteoarthritis and indications for total knee arthroplasty for general practitioners. J Am Osteopath Assoc.2012; 112(11):709-15.
22. Rankin EA, Alarcon GS, Chang RW, Cooney Jr LM, Costley LS, Delitto A, et al. NIH consensus statement on total knee replacement. 2003.
23. Kane R, Saleh K, Wilt TJ, Bershadsky B, Cross WW, MacDonald RM, et al. Total knee replacement. Evidence report/technology assessment. 2005.
24. Health Quality Ontario. Total knee replacement: an evidence-based analysis. 2005. 5(9): 1-51.
25. Total Knee Replacement - Ontario Health Technology Assessment Series 2005;5(9).
26. Total Knee Replacement. American Academy of Orthopedic Surgeons. 2011.
27. Minimally invasive total knee arthroplasty for osteoarthritis. N Engl J Med. 2009;360 (17):1749-58. .
28. Motohashi M, Adachi A, et al. Deep vein thrombosis in orthopedic surgery of the lower extremities. Annals of Vascular Diseases. 2012; 5(3): 328-33.
29. Leone JM, Hanssen AD..Management of infection at the site of a total knee arthroplasty. 2006.
30. Kerkhoffs GM, Servien E, Dunn W, Dahm D, Bramer JA, Haverkamp D. The influence of obesity on the complication rate and outcome of total knee arthroplasty: a meta-analysis and systematic literature review. The Journal of Bone and Joint Surgery. 2012;94(20):1839-44.
31. Samson AJ, Mercer GE, Campbell DG. Total knee replacement in the morbidly obese: a literature review. 2010.
32. Subotnick SI. Return to sport after delayed surgical reconstruction for ankle instability. In: Nyska, M, Mann, G (Eds). The Unstable Ankle. Human Kinetics, Champaign, IL, 2002, pp. 201-5.

Index

Page numbers followed by *f* refer to figure.